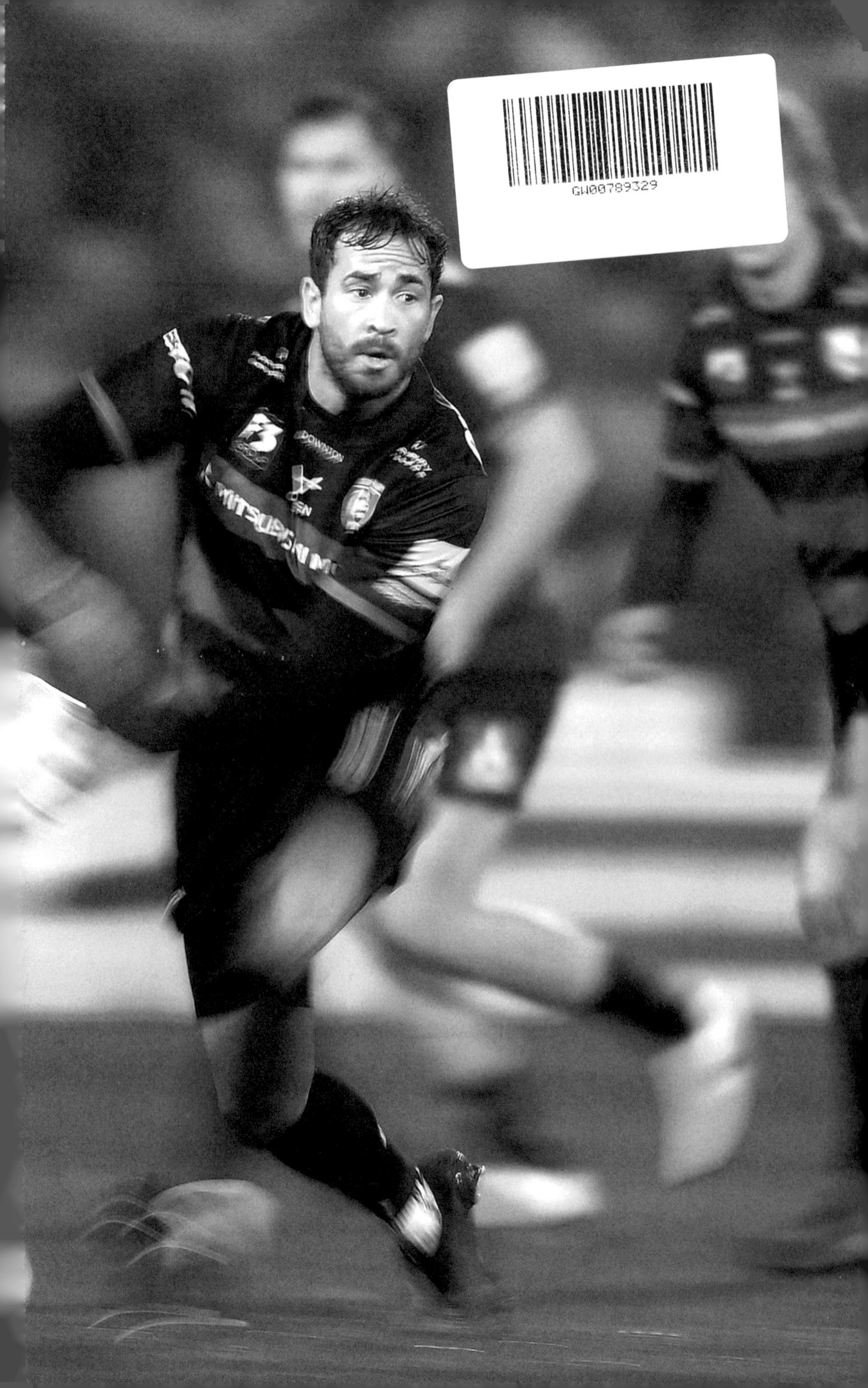
GW00789329

DANNY CIPRIANI

WHO AM I?

HarperCollins*Publishers*

I dedicate this book to my wonderful wife Victoria Rose. The journey we have been on is nothing short of remarkable. We have walked and danced with each other's demons and in return made it safe for us to deal with them ourselves. You are my favourite chapter and one that remains open with many pages left to fill, we were always meant to be together. It was only ever you. It will only ever be you. You are the most special and beautiful woman I've ever met in my life. Every bit of pain, every wrong decision, every moment of despair, now feels necessary and entirely worth it with you by my side. You have inspired me to be the best possible man I could be, your love set me free. With you I now know what eternity feels like. God sure did take his time with you. Love you.

I also dedicate this book to anyone wanting to transform themselves, to the people who do not have hope, to the people who are sensitive, to the people who don't fit in, to the people who feel like they are repeatedly banging their head on a brick wall, to the people who want to feel better but may be going down a wrong path, to the people avoiding those tough and dark areas that are too painful to face, to the people who feel unloved or unseen, to the people putting on a brave face every day, to the people numbing or distracting your mind. I salute you. There is a power within you that you may not recognise yet. Take the step of faith for yourself. Learn yourself. Be kind to yourself. Forgive yourself. Love yourself.

HarperCollins*Publishers*
1 London Bridge Street
London SE1 9GF

www.harpercollins.co.uk

HarperCollins*Publishers*
Macken House, 39/40 Mayor Street Upper
Dublin 1, D01 C9W8, Ireland

First published by HarperCollins*Publishers* 2023

1 3 5 7 9 10 8 6 4 2

A catalogue record of this book is
available from the British Library

HB ISBN 978-0-00-861728-8

Printed and bound in the UK using 100%
renewable electricity at CPI Group (UK) Ltd

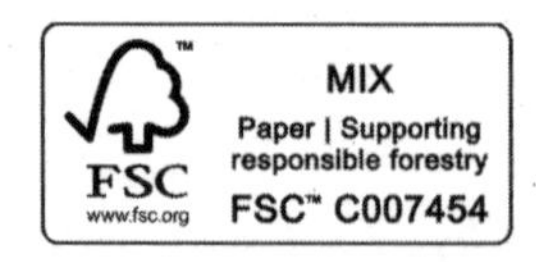

This book is produced from independently certified FSC™ paper
to ensure responsible forest management.

For more information visit: www.harpercollins.co.uk/green

CONTENTS

Prologue

SO MUCH SWEETER

I was planning on finding out the truth when Mum stayed for Christmas – but she still wasn't ready to give up her secrets. I'd ask questions, she wouldn't respond, and eventually I'd give up.

I drove Mum home on 27 December. And now it was just me and her, I thought I'd give it one last shot. It was the same as before, like bashing my head against a brick wall. But instead of getting frustrated, I thought to myself, *You know what? Maybe I don't need answers*, and held her hand instead.

We were still holding hands when I pulled up at Mum's house 25 minutes later. She turned to me and said, 'That's the best thing you could have done.'

On New Year's Eve, Mum's friend called to say she hadn't heard from her for three days, and that something must be up. Me and my wife Victoria jumped in the car, drove to Mum's house and found her slumped on the sofa.

At the hospital, they told us she'd suffered a stroke. Now, I'd never know the answers to all those questions. *Why does it have to be this way between us? Why all the lies?* But the only thing that matters, for me and for Mum, is that she sees how much I love her.

The ward Mum's in is like God's waiting room. All the other patients are stroke victims but a lot older than her – she's only in her early sixties. They're covered in cuts and bruises because they keep falling over. Not a great place for anyone to get better. No wonder Mum is convinced she's going to die.

I've had to speak to her about power of attorney, so I can take care of everything she'll need when she eventually comes to live with me and Victoria – her own special chair, an adapted bedroom and toilet. It must be scary giving up all your information, because it's almost an admission you don't have long left. And Mum's never been good at sharing things with me.

Luckily, being like Mum has its advantages. Yes, she's got an almighty battle on her hands, but inside that rickety exterior is a core of steel. I know, because I've been trying to reach it for as long as I can remember.

When the stroke happened, on New Year's Eve 2022, me and Victoria thought Mum might never walk or talk again. Then one day, Mum said her first words to me: 'You are weird.' Not so long ago, that would have cut me deep. But I just smiled, because I now know that my job as a son is to give her my love unconditionally, which I suspect she's never experienced.

Eight weeks later, she got out of her chair and walked to the toilet unaided. She's got a bit of a gangster lean and is slow and unsteady on her feet – I suspect she'll need a pimp stick at some point – but she's a million miles from where she was.

The doctors say the stroke triggered dementia, so she's said one or two unfortunate things to the nurses. But it also seems to have opened her up emotionally. On one of my first visits, I could see she wanted to say something. I leaned in and said, 'Mum, whatever you've got to say, don't worry about it. It's been and gone.' She replied, in not much more than a whisper, 'I'm trying my best to be a decent mum.' She looked brighter, as if a cloud had lifted.

There's beauty in everything if you strive to make yourself aware of it. And since Mum's stroke, our relationship has been better than ever. Some days, she even cuddles me before I leave, and there are glimpses of affection, which is not something I've ever experienced. The emotion bubbles over sometimes, but I know it's better to lift her spirits.

While Victoria can't comprehend how calm I've been, it hasn't surprised me. I can still remember what it felt like to be chasing all the time, the chaos and the speed of it. I had to drink and take prescription drugs to slow things down. But I've reached a point where I can happily sit quietly on my own in silence for hours, with no thoughts in my head. That's when I feel an almost spiritual presence.

There's been a lot of nonsense written about me, but lately I've been getting social media messages along the lines of, 'I'm just so happy you're happy.'

It's true, I am happy, and I wish everyone could feel like I do. But it's taken a lot of self-reflection and honesty. I've been searching for the real me for most of my life, and most of that time I was groping in the dark – unless I was on a rugby field. Only recently, through my experiences and discoveries, have I learned to accept that darkness and start living in a brighter present.

Not long ago I spoke at the Oxford Union, which was ironic because Mum was still telling me to go to university after I'd played for England. Before I went, I said to her, 'You always wanted me to go to Oxford, well now I'm going. And I didn't even have to apply.' Because I didn't want to force anything or deliver a speech, which would have taken me out of the moment, which is where I want to be, I spoke freely and without fear of judgement. My body came over all prickly while I was speaking, but that prickliness wasn't nerves, it came from stepping into the new, the thrill of saying the truth and facing the feeling of not belonging.

A lot of this stuff has been swirling around in my head for a long time, but it would have been a different book had I written it just a few years ago, full of pain and resistance. Still, dredging up all the trauma from my past has brought out emotions I didn't know I had in me, because I didn't deal with it at the time.

But I've learned that I can't always be Danny Cipriani who played rugby, partly because hardly anyone will remember that I did in 20 years' time, partly because that's a reductive way of thinking, a sure way of restricting my growth. It would be tragic if I decided that playing for England was the pinnacle of my life when I still might have 50 years to live.

Rest easy, I'm not going to claim I was some kind of angel and people didn't notice my halo. I'm not even going to follow that sentence with a 'but'.

What I will say is that telling the truth is a whole lot better than allowing other people to control the narrative, people who wanted everyone to think I was one of the worst human beings ever to walk the earth. A misfit, a malcontent, a sub-human scum. They were so convincing, even I believed them.

If I hold stuff back, don't reveal how I felt at my lowest and highest points, then it will be impossible for the reader to understand how I've reached the point I have now. To that end, I thought it was important to describe events as I was feeling then, not as I'm feeling today. So you'll find frustration, anger, despair and regret in the coming pages. You'll see the chaos of my mind, while I was chasing my needs and desires, when I was acting impulsively and never really listening to myself. You'll feel my peace, when I was on a rugby field, free of thought, just being. It might upset a few people. But I never set out to belittle anyone, or sell anyone out, it's just what happened.

Maybe if I was sitting here with 100 England caps to my name, I'd be an insufferable braggart and the next few hundred pages would mainly be about how wonderful I've been for the last however many years. As it is, the fact that not everything went my way means I got what I needed to face the parts of me I'd been running from.

I was about as low as it's possible to be but got through it and emerged into a magical place. Because that's what my life is now. Everything's flowing right, I'm peaceful, full of love and free, just trying to play what's in front of me.

But there's one thing I've always known, even when it was buried among the rubble of my mind: it's better to follow your heart and be true to yourself than play by other people's rules. You might not be accepted by everyone, and it will be more painful, but the rewards, when they finally come, will be so much sweeter than any trophy.

1

NOT THE DANNY I KNEW

I want to be seen. But not like this. Every time I make eye contact with someone, I imagine they're thinking horrible things. Something they've read on the internet, seen on TV or heard their friend say. *What about that Danny Cipriani? What an idiot, had the world at his feet and chucked it all away.*

I pass an old guy sitting on a bench. He closes his newspaper, lowers his glasses and follows me like a portrait in a gallery. A young bloke double-takes, elbows his girlfriend in the ribs and hisses, 'That's Cipriani ...' He thinks he's being subtle – or maybe he doesn't. Either way, I can hear it from the other side of the road, followed by the mocking laughter of his girlfriend.

I pick up the pace, so that I'm virtually trotting. Head down, the peak of my cap pulled almost over my eyes. I'd say I was skulking, but it's not possible to skulk when you're in the tabloids every day, hardly ever for the right reasons, and when you're radiating gloom, which is visible from miles away.

I cross the roundabout, enter the little corner shop, which is busier than I hoped it would be, and head straight for the counter. A woman with a little boy looks at me and smiles. But before she can say anything to me – and I can tell she wants to say something to me – I order a bottle of vodka. The man behind the counter plonks the bottle down and names the price. He probably has no idea who I am, but his eyes say to me, *Take your vodka and get out of here*. As I'm leaving, I hear the woman say, 'Do you know who that was?'

I hide the bottle up my jumper and scurry home. It's only a two-minute walk but it's a race against time, before the walls close in and squash me.

Back in the house, I plonk myself on the sofa, pour myself a drink and take a long swig. For the rest of the day, it's just me and my vodka. I've never felt so alone.

If I sound paranoid, that's because I am. I feel picked to pieces, like the whole world has turned against me, thinks I'm a wrong 'un, a suspicious character.

You know what I read the other day? *What the hell has Cipriani got to be unhappy about? Plays rugby for a living, good-looking bloke, shagged half the women in Britain. That boy needs to find some perspective.* But it's not like I can say to myself, *Snap out of it, Danny, think how handsome you are!* That kind of stuff is irrelevant when your mind is churning over thoughts like mine. And it's difficult to have perspective when you're scrabbling around in the gutter, desperately trying to locate a few crumbs of self-worth.

Journalists seem to think the words they write are harmless. But they do real damage. As for the readers, they look at my life – at the glamorous women, the nice restaurants I eat in, the expensive car that keeps getting tickets – and think everything is shiny. But I feel like an experiment – *Let's send this kid out into the unforgiving, judgemental world and see what happens to him.* I've even started believing what the papers keep writing: that I'm one of the worst people on the planet, giving Gaddafi and Bin Laden a run for their money.

Halfway down the bottle and it just gets murkier. When I first arrived on the scene, I could do almost nothing wrong. I'd play okay and they'd write that I played brilliantly. I'd play well and they'd write that I was some kind of genius. Only two years ago, they were calling me the saviour of English rugby, a new hero, a prince even – ushering in a New Jerusalem. Not sure what that meant, but it sounded great. They wanted a hero, and for a while I was it.

Now I'm thinking about that game against Ireland in 2008. Man, did I get England cooking that day. I was seeing pictures no-one else was seeing. But there was nothing flash about it, it was just common sense to me. Making the right decisions, creating space, getting the different parts flowing as one. Architecture, if you like, on the hoof. To do that, your brain has to work as fast as your hands and your feet. But it felt effortless, like it was the only thing I'd been put on this earth to do.

But the success I'd desperately been trying to achieve since I was a little kid, and the joy it brought, was fleeting.

I've been chasing that feeling ever since and never caught up with it. And it seems like such a long time ago. That 20-year-old kid, so bubbly and high on life, is nothing but a fuzzy memory.

All I ever wanted was to play for England, but the only people I want to be seen by, the England coaches, have put on the blinkers. The door to that world has been slammed shut and double bolted. Now, I'm the fifth-choice fly-half in the country. Or is it the sixth? I've stopped counting. England wouldn't have me ushering in the half-time oranges, let alone a New Jerusalem.

Now when I play okay for my club, journalists write that I played badly. When I play well, they write that I played okay, but should have done better. There are stories about me having a bad attitude, slinking in and slinking out again without talking to anyone. They claim my team-mates want me gone.

Somewhere down the line, the narrative changed. But I'm still the same player, can still do things other players can't. That seems obvious to me, but the people who matter aren't seeing it. Rugby in this country isn't honest. I think that even when I'm sober and thinking straight.

I've even thought about quitting rugby and doing something else, because it feels like a job I hate, something that has been corrupted. Paradoxically, the only place I really find peace is on the rugby field. On the field, my brain stops ticking over, because I'm just doing the thing I love.

* * *

This vodka certainly isn't giving me peace. It's just making my brain produce negative thoughts at a faster rate. Thing is, I can't blame everyone else, I have to hold my hands up, take some responsibility for the situation I'm in.

Maybe they're right and all the fame has gone to my head, ruined me as a person and a player. But that just makes me feel worse. It's easier if you can pin the blame on other people. That way, you don't feel as much regret.

People in rugby know my head's not right, and hasn't been right for ages, but there's not much emotional intelligence in the game. You leave a team, or get cut adrift, and you just have to cope. But I'm not coping. I can't see any future, I can't see any hope. I feel like I've got nothing to live for.

I peak through the curtains, looking for paparazzi. Those fuckers will follow you to the ends of the earth to get a snap of you at your lowest ebb. They've been lurking outside for months, snapping me putting out the bins, removing tickets from my car windscreen. Stuff readers of the tabloids are apparently dying to see. If they're lucky, they'll get a picture of us together, the perfect celebrity package – even though one of us never wanted to be a celebrity. They'll get a couple of pages out of that, and presumably a fair few grand – 'Rugby's Bad Boy and the Sexiest Woman in Britain.' And if anyone questions their intrusion, they'll say, 'They're famous, what's the issue?'

My girlfriend's beautiful, there's no getting away from that. But that woman you see in the papers, posing in her underwear, every man's fantasy, isn't doing me much good. One minute, everything's great. The next, she wants to tear it all up. And she doesn't seem interested in how things are affecting me. That's not great when you have no-one else to lean on, when your dad deserted you years ago and your mum thinks everything she reads is gospel.

Part of me knows this relationship isn't real, but she's convinced me it's us against the world, that we're safer together. And I don't have the courage to finish things and face the inevitable media and public backlash. So we carry on.

When I finally decided to end it all, I went through the options. I thought about overdosing on pills, but what if I survived and ended up brain dead? I'd still be here but just a drain on other people. I thought about jumping off a tall building but decided that would give me too much time to change my mind.

That's why I thought a gun would be best. Aim it at my head, pull the trigger, BOOM! A quick way to bring all this pain to an end. I've decided not to leave a note, so that people can draw their own conclusions. I'm sure they'll say, 'He seemed to have the perfect life. A mystery. Doesn't make sense.'

If the man with the gun turns up today, I'll go through with it. He's just some guy I met in the West End. Naughty boy, fancies himself as a gangster, asks no questions. Problem is, I keep changing my mind and he's starting to get annoyed, like gangsters, plastic or otherwise, tend to do.

I message him again. This time, I say, I really am serious. A few minutes later, the doorbell rings. I take another peak through the curtains, but it's not the man with the gun, it's my mate Ed. I'd forgotten he was paying me a visit.

I take Ed through to the living room and we sit next to each other on the sofa. He asks me how I am and I tell him I'm fine. But the almost empty bottle of vodka tells him I'm not. We exchange a bit of idle chat and I think I'm coming across as normal. No tears, and I certainly don't tell him about the gun. I don't want anyone to know, in case they try to talk me out of it.

But the more we speak, the more I'm aware that Ed can feel my darkness. He's known me far too long. The conversation grinds to a halt and there's a gaping, uncomfortable silence. Then Ed turns to me and says, 'Mate, this isn't you. This is not the Danny I knew when we were kids.'

2

PART OF MY HEART

I'm nine years old and the most confident person out here. Dads sound tense on the touchline, which is rubbing off on some of the kids. Meanwhile, I'm thinking, *Let's get this game underway. We can handle it!*

The whistle goes, they kick off and one of our forwards catches the ball. He knows what to do. He passes to the scrum-half, who passes it to me. I drop the shoulder, step on the gas, swerve outside the defender and score under the posts. This is freedom. This is joy. This is living gloriously in the moment.

Even before I get the ball, I'm working things out and excited by the possibilities. *Pass inside? Long pass out wide? Little chip through? Sod it, let's go outside again and score myself.* To me, a rugby field is like an adventure playground. A place to explore, get into mischief. Have fun!

The other team's coach is getting agitated. Their dads are shouting stuff from the touchline. None of it makes sense, because they don't know rugby like they think they do. And they're injecting all their nonsense into their kids, instead of letting them discover things for themselves. The way they're talking – 'Hit him early!' 'Hit him high!' 'Hit him low!' – you'd think tackling me was easy. I feel like saying, 'Why don't you put some boots on and try it yourself?'

I get the ball behind our posts and shape to pass, before stepping the other way and leaving the tackler in the splits position. Where others would see a wall of players, I see space. I pull out a skip-step I've learned from players on the telly, leave two more tacklers grasping at thin air, kick cross-field, and our winger scoops up the ball on the run and scores in the corner.

I look over at our dads cheering and clapping on the touchline. But mine's not there.

Mum and Dad met at a party in Tobago. The following day, Dad saw Mum on the beach, ran up behind her and lifted her in the air. Isn't it funny how things happen? If Mum hadn't gone to the beach that day – maybe she had a headache from the party or went shopping instead – I might not be here.

They must have liked each other quite a lot, because Dad moved over from Tobago, they got married and Mum got pregnant. But I don't remember anything about the good times, because they split up when I was two.

Dad lives north of the river – Willesden, Harlesden, Hammersmith, wherever he lays his hat – while I live with Mum on the Lockyer estate in Putney, on the fifth floor of a block of flats. Mostly she works, she says, to get money to give me everything I want. Or she tells me how much she hates my dad. But sometimes I just want a hug and a kiss. Or just for her to see me.

Mum drives a black cab, which is quite unusual for a woman. She's out the door before I get up for school, gets home around 4 p.m. to make me dinner, then goes back out again until just before I go to bed. She wanted Dad to do the Knowledge, too, so that he could drive a cab and earn good money. But Dad likes to drink, and drinking and driving a cab don't go together too well.

Dad's very different to Mum, probably because he's from the Caribbean. He tells me that growing up in Trinidad, where he lived before moving to Tobago, everything was more relaxed. 'Danny,' he says. 'Life wasn't about getting a job, getting a mortgage, always chasing – it was how quickly can I get to the beach and do nothing all day.'

That sounds like a great life – being free, doing what you want – and I'm not saying it's wrong. But in London, he does have to get a job and a mortgage. He does have to chase things, because he's got me to look after on weekends.

Mum's the serious parent and Dad's the fun one. When I'm with him, I feel happy and free, safe and loved. That's maybe why I feel more black than white, even though most people don't realise I'm black at all.

Dad taught me to swim at nine months old, which he seems incredibly proud of, and is a really good instructor, brilliant with kids. When he does lessons at Acton Baths, sometimes I'll join in, but usually I'll be messing about on the side. After swimming, Dad takes me to the Irish pub.

When we walk in, people slap him on the back and ruffle my hair. Everyone knows me as Jay's son, and they all seem to love me.

Sometimes, Dad talks about how much he hates my mum. But he also talks about nice stuff, like his ancestors in Trinidad. Between gulps of Guinness, he tells stories about 'Marvellous' Mikey Cipriani, Trinidad's greatest ever athlete and famous aviator; or Captain Cipriani, the heroic labour leader and politician. There's a Cipriani Boulevard in Port of Spain, and a statue of Captain Cipriani in Independence Square. Dad says the Ciprianis were originally from Corsica and were closely related to the Bonaparte family, as in Napoleon. I don't know if that's true or not, but I'm running with it.

When I was a toddler, Dad had a bad accident – he was hit by a drunk-driver while riding his moped – and had a metal bar inserted in his leg. As a result, he struggles with the English weather, especially in the winter. So sometimes, he talks about how he'd like to go home to Tobago. When that comes up, I try not to listen.

We're not always in the pub, sometimes we play cricket. I started playing for Dad's team, which is made up of blokes from all over the Caribbean, when I was eight or nine, and my goal every time is to score more runs than him. He fancies himself as another Brian Lara, but I started outscoring Dad when I was nine. I give him so much shit for that.

One week, I pull off the most ridiculous catch, sticking out a hand and somehow managing to drag the ball in from almost behind me. Everyone's looking at each other as if to say, 'What the hell have I just seen?' Later, Dad's mate Roger keels over with a heart attack. Dad tells me to stay with him and keep him on his side, and when Roger recovers, he says I saved his life.

Dad also takes me to play football for Acton Ealing Whistlers. I'm pretty handy, and QPR and Chelsea seem to be interested in signing me. But when I get a scholarship to a private prep school, rugby just naturally takes over.

Just because you get a scholarship, that doesn't mean you don't have to pay anything. For starters, I've got to catch the 93 bus every day, from Putney to Wimbledon. Then there's the uniform, school activities and what not. Mum drives that cab all hours and we live in a council house. But she still has to pay for food and bills, so I'm not too sure how she scrapes the money together.

The rugby coach at Donhead Prep is an Irishman called Mr O'Dea. He's a tough guy, a disciplinarian who takes no nonsense. But he's also funny, with a lightness about him. For some reason, he's always really nice to me and talking me up in front of other people.

At the end of Monday assembly, he reads the weekend's sports results. It's always quite formal, until he gets to my team. Then he'll say something like, And Little Red Booty Boy scored four tries again. In case you're wondering, Little Red Booty Boy is me. Mr O'Dea makes me feel like I'm worth something and I think the world of him. I certainly never want to let him down.

Maybe the best thing about Mr O'Dea is how he lets me be who I want to be on the rugby field. He doesn't bang on about tactics, he wants us to run free and express ourselves.

One game, between Donhead and Dulwich Prep, I take a tap penalty and throw the ball, American football style, to the opposite wing, where my team-mate catches it and scores a try. Like Mr O'Dea often says, 'If you think something is the best thing to do, don't hesitate, just do it.' When I look over at Mr O'Dea on the touchline, he's got a little smile on his face.

Afterwards, this well-spoken dad, whose son plays for Dulwich, comes over to me and my mum, introduces himself as Roger Hamilton-Brown and asks if I'd like to play for Rosslyn Park. I've never heard of Rosslyn Park, but this bloke's not just well-spoken, he sounds almost royal, so I say, 'Yeah, sounds cool.'

Turns out Roger has been scouting players at various tournaments for weeks, because he's assembling a crack team of 10-year-olds. Roger drives me and his son Rory to games in his Bentley. He'll be bombing it down the hard shoulder and say, 'Listen boys, if the police pull us over, one of you pretend you're sick and I'll say I'm rushing to hospital.' He even buys me some new boots. I assume he does that because he sees how talented and keen I am.

But I reckon he also sees something different in me, a wildness that can perhaps be harnessed, a playful abandon the other kids don't have. I don't suppose they spend much time down the pub with their dads.

One of my team-mates is a black kid called Neville Edwards, whose mum is from Trinidad and Tobago. When I first meet him and tell him my dad is from Trinidad as well, he gives me a funny look. Only after I fill him in on the details does he believe me, and we become best of friends.

One day, Dad turns up to our flat in Putney, out of the blue. He isn't there long, just enough time to tell me he's going home to Tobago. For good.

'The taxi's outside,' he says. 'I have to go now.'

I don't know what to say. But as he walks out the door, something clicks. I go flying after him, but by the time I've reached the landing, the lift doors are closing. I tear down the stairs, bawling my eyes out, intercept him as he's leaving the lift and grab his leg. I'm holding onto his leg, pleading for him to stay, all the way to the taxi. Part of my heart is torn out that day.

3

AT LEAST I'M FREE

When Dad went home, part of Mum left, too. It's not like everything's suddenly gone to shit and me and Mum are constantly at each other's throats. But she's even colder than she was before. All work and no play.

Mum's been carrying a great burden since splitting with Dad – that burden being me. I know she feels unable to live a life of her own, because she often tells me that everything she does, she does for me. As such, I'm also carrying a great burden. And I still can't find a way to her heart.

There are photos of Mum hugging me and smiling, but I can't remember those times. And I have this horrible feeling we'll never get back there.

Luckily, there are lots of other kids to hang about with on the Lockyer estate. I spend whole days playing football in the metal cage around the back. I'm the youngest, but because I'm good, the older kids want me in their team.

We get up to some mischief, but nothing really horrible. The worst thing I've done is steal from Mrs Thompson's sweet shop behind the pub. I knew poor old Mrs Thompson was slow on her feet, so I nicked a chocolate bar and legged it. I felt so bad, I ran back in, put 50p on the counter and ran off again.

I'm starting to see more kids from the neighbouring estate, which can only spell trouble. Not long ago, I went on a bike ride and when we got to the other estate, this kid picked up a brick and threw it through a window. We all started pedalling like mad, but when I jumped off a kerb, my wheel buckled and I went over the handlebars. Luckily, one of the big kids came back, picked me up and backied me home.

I'm not exactly living the thug life, but Mum decides to send me off to boarding school when I'm 11. Something to do with her mum being ill, which I just accept as gospel. It's another scholarship, but it still costs money, which means Mum's working more than ever.

I don't have any of those boarding school horror stories you hear about, like being made to eat soggy biscuits or prefects using my arse as a toast rack. Reading Oratory is mostly great, because I get to play sport every day.

There's rugby, football, cricket, tennis, squash, whatever takes my fancy. And because I'm good at sport, I don't have any problems fitting in. My sporting talent gives me confidence, a social cachet, respect. Even most of the adults treat me differently to other students, almost with reverence.

The season I score 36 goals in 12 games, Reading FC send a coach to watch me six or seven times, and there's some talk about me signing youth forms. And on the cricket field, I'm scoring so many runs at the age of 12 that they put me in the first team, with 18-year-olds. But after two years at boarding school, I want out.

I'm spending a ridiculous amount of time travelling every weekend. And while I don't feel abandoned, I do feel like I'm in the wrong place. It's not really my culture, which is the rough and tumble of the Lockyer estate.

Plus, my two best mates from Rosslyn Park, Nev and Adam Thompstone, keep telling me great things about Whitgift, which is one of the best rugby schools in the country. I imagine a rugby team with me, Nev and Adam in it would be unbeatable, so I beg Mum to bring me home. In the end, she caves and agrees to send me to Whitgift instead.

I feel right at home at Whitgift. It's a private school, but very diverse. There are loads of kids from poorer backgrounds on scholarships and bursaries, like me and Nev, and there's a mix of ethnicities, because it's bang in the middle of Croydon. At Whitgift, it's not about money, it's about excellence, creating as many opportunities as possible for pupils to fulfil their potential. And I feel like everyone, from Dr Barnet the headmaster down, is on my side (apart from the odd teacher who values academia over sport and sees me as a cocky so and so).

I could do without the schoolwork, can't see how it's relevant. If a teacher respects me, I put more effort in. And if a teacher is hot, I'll be on my best behaviour.

When Rosslyn Park tour South Africa, my programme profile reads, 'He's a talented sportsman who is always keen to hear the coach's opinion.' Whoever wrote that was being sarcastic, because often I do the opposite of what the coach says. And they don't mind, because it usually comes off.

When you're doing brilliant things every time you step on to a sporting field, the adulation grows and so does your ego. I have an unshakeable belief in myself on a rugby, football or cricket field. It's the place I love, and where I feel free and seen.

But while I make the odd joke about my talent, no-one would describe me as in-your-face cocky. And if it sometimes looks like I'm trying to do everything on my own, it's not because I'm showing off – *Look at me! Look at how great I am!* – it's because I think it's best for the team.

Nev tells me some of the boys are moaning because I never pass to them. They're right, in that they don't get the ball as much as Nev or Adam, but that's just because we're on the same page. I'm not trying to belittle anyone, I'm just doing what needs to be done.

Truth be told, I've always enjoyed creating tries for team-mates far more than scoring them myself. There's something more fulfilling about that.

The last few summer holidays, I've visited Dad in Tobago. Everyone on Dad's side is black, so they love it when this little white boy turns up. I suppose I'm a novelty, but I'm never made to feel as if I'm not part of the family. My gran, Dad's mum, is crazy strict with my cousins. If they step out of line, she'll scream at them and give them a whack. But she lets me do whatever I like.

When I'm over there, I can see why Dad came home. He's right, everything is more relaxed. But now I'm a bit older, I'm wondering how Dad gets by. I see what he means about not chasing anything in Tobago, and how nice it feels to do nothing on the beach all day, but I also know that adults need to work to get money. If there's one thing Mum's taught me, it's that.

I'm often on one of Dad's boat tours, and even then he'll have a bottle of Carib lager in hand. He'll be holding court, dancing around, making the tourists laugh. Maybe he's the wise one, because he seems happy enough.

Everyone knows my dad, because Tobago's not a big place and he's usually the loudest in the room. Or on the beach. So while I get a few double-takes the first time I'm there, from people wondering why this white kid is hanging out with the locals, it soon feels like home to me. People shout, 'Hey, Danny boy!' Everything feels easy and comfortable and nice.

One day, when I'm 14, I'm asked to play for a men's team, as in an actual league match in front of about 200 people. I score with my left foot, another with my right, before completing my hat-trick with a header. People are losing their minds. One bloke bolts from the crowd, picks me up and starts running around the pitch. He must think he's discovered the white Dwight Yorke.

But now I've had a few new father figures to look up to – serious, responsible men, like Mr O'Dea – I have a different take on those days down the Irish pub, watching Dad drink Guinness and listening to his stories, or those idyllic days in Tobago, watching Dad do much the same on the beach.

I look at some of my mate's dads, the ones who are always getting riled up on the touchline, and I'm glad my dad's not like them. Yeah, I'm lonely, but at least I'm not scared stiff of disappointing anyone but myself. At least I'm free.

NEVILLE EDWARDS

When we were kids, people would say to me, 'Danny can't be black, his skin's too light.' I'd have to convince them his dad was from Trinidad, like my mum. And it was that shared heritage that made us so close from the get-go.

Dan was a likeable, happy-go-lucky kid, and very good at whatever sport he turned his hand to. But because he was so talented, and able to see things that others couldn't, including his coaches, he was also challenging.

He'd always ask questions: 'Why are we doing it that way? Can we do it this way instead?' If they said no, he'd do it his way anyway. And nine times out of ten, his way would work.

I'm sure some coaches weren't happy about being overruled by a kid, but he wasn't doing it to be disruptive, he just wanted to get better. Although I didn't see that at the time, because I didn't have Dan's sporting intelligence.

Opposition players and disgruntled parents of team-mates who weren't getting picked would call Dan cocky or arrogant, but I thought he was just very confident in his own ability. Often, he'd tell you what he was going to do and then do it. And if you questioned him, he could take it badly.

One game for Rosslyn Park, when we were 11 or 12, we had a falling out. We'd been given a penalty on the halfway line, and everyone was telling him to kick to the corner, but he was adamant he could slot the three points. After some toing and froing, I grabbed the ball, pushed it into his chest and said, 'Just do whatever you want.' He kicked to the corner, and after we'd scored a try from the line-out, he said to me, 'Don't ever tell me what to do.'

A few minutes later, we got a penalty from the same spot as before, and this time Dan wasn't discussing it. Sure enough, his kick sailed between the posts. And, to be fair to Dan, we had a laugh about it afterwards.

Dan did ridiculous things every game he played. If we were in a close game, he'd be that kid who said, 'Just give me the ball.' His speciality was the chip and chase, which almost always worked a treat. He'd kick the ball over the top, it would usually sit up perfectly, and either me or him would latch on to it and score. I scored a lot of tries because of Dan, including the two he set up for me when Whitgift won the national schools under-15 cup final at Twickenham. Mighty Millfield were favourites that day, but we beat them comfortably.

Dan was always a step ahead of his team-mates, but when he joined the National Academy, he went to another level. He wasn't just playing anymore, he was managing games, and his skillset was far wider. You could tell he'd been practising and practising, because he was nailing everything.

I was let go by London Irish when I was 18, which was devastating. I went to university, got a normal job and returned to

Rosslyn Park, who were in the third tier of English rugby. But I never gave up hope of playing in the Premiership. Then when Dan was at Sale, he arranged a trial for me. I quit my job, trained my arse off, did pre-season for free and ended up getting a contract.

I was Sale's top try-scorer in my first season, and a lot of that was down to Dan. I'd always done extras after training, and now I was a full-time pro, I did even more. Me and Dan did a lot of stuff together, and he wouldn't just teach me the basics, it was technical stuff no coach had even mentioned before, mainly to do with kicking and positioning, in attack and defence. And after I'd showered and changed, Dan would still be out on the training ground. Some days, he'd be out there on his own for hours.

Dan's attention to detail was forensic, but he wasn't always great at articulating his thoughts. He could have been softer at times, but when you're in a high-pressure sporting environment, and you need to make quick decisions, you sometimes need to be blunt. Besides, all healthy workplaces have conflict, because only when people are challenged do they get better.

Dan became more nuanced over time – he'd speak to some players more gently than others – which is why he'd be a great coach, because he's got the emotional intelligence to go with his deep understanding of the game.

It was strange reading all that negative stuff about him in the media. There were things he could have done differently, for sure, but I knew what he was really like, which was very far from how they portrayed him.

I also found the England situation bonkers. Dan had so much to give, and he really wanted to give it. It was tough seeing how hard he worked, how excited he was about playing for his country, and still getting rejected.

But my biggest beef with England was their lack of honesty, which is a problem with rugby in general, because it's such a macho environment. If they'd been up front about it, told Dan that he was never going to fit in with how they wanted to play the game, he wouldn't have been happy, but at least he'd have known where he stood. As it was, he'd sometimes say to me, 'Why am I not getting a shot, Nev?' And he never really got any answers.

Back then, we spoke more about our frustrations than our deeper feelings, which is common among male friends. But I could see how much it hurt him, as it would have hurt anyone. I just hoped he'd stand toe to toe with adversity, rather than fold and go under. Thankfully, that's what happened.

4

PLAY THE GAME

I was leaning towards playing cricket for Surrey because I love batting so much. It's me versus 11 other blokes, but really it's me versus me. And when I get my eye in, there are few better feelings. I've scored a few tons and once hit 50 from 18 balls, but I've decided to play rugby for England instead.

Rosslyn Park haven't lost for years. I reckon between me, Rory, Adam and Nev, we'd have one of the fastest 4x100m relay quartets in the country.

I don't take too well to instruction, probably because I've never had much at home. But what's great about Rosslyn Park is that the coaches let the players do what they want and trust them to come up trumps on the day.

If they tell me to do something, I'll listen. But when I'm on the field, their instructions go out of the window. They're cool with that. They understand that it's us playing the game, and we're a free-spirited group of lads.

I listen to some of the stuff opposition coaches shout from the touchline and it's obvious they don't know what they're talking about. You can tell some of them have only watched rugby on TV, and they're probably not watching the best stuff. Me, I'm watching club rugby from down under every weekend, and I love the Hurricanes from Wellington.

The Hurricanes backline is ridiculous, particularly their full-back Christian Cullen. The way he runs, he reminds me of a stone skipping over the surface of a lake. He's got several gears, a wicked swerve, can leave a defender for dead off both feet, and his timing into the line is almost always perfect.

I'll often think, I know who'd win between the Hurricanes and the best club team in England. And it wouldn't be much of a contest.

I think the people who slag off Super Rugby are very narrow-minded. Rugby can be played in many different ways, as people like Christian Cullen prove. Our players can't do what their players do, so people pretend they're not playing the same game. But they are. They're just playing it better.

For a long time, sport was just about having fun with my mates. I knew I was good, and I loved the competition, but I couldn't imagine something so enjoyable could be my life. But the rugby's started to get more serious, which means I've had to knock the football and cricket on the head. Goodbye Wembley, farewell Lord's, it's full steam ahead to Twickenham.

When I'm 15, I start doing bits and bobs with Wasps and get called up to the RFU's Junior National Academy three years early. I knew I was a decent player but seeing that England rose on the letterhead was mind-blowing. It was like receiving a letter from Father Christmas, instead of the other way around.

The same year, I play for England Under-16s and win the national schools under-15 cup with Whitgift, setting up two tries for Nev. I feel right at home at Twickenham because I've been playing there for various teams since I was 10.

I've been looking in the mirror for ages, admiring my England tracksuit. I run my fingers over the embroidered red rose and can't help smiling. Just a few years ago, I was booting a football about in a cage on the Lockyer estate. Now, I'm wearing the same gear as Jonny Wilkinson when he won the World Cup.

The manager of the National Academy is Brian Ashton, who used to coach Bath and work under England head coach Clive Woodward. But even though he's coached all sorts of star players, from Jeremy Guscott at Bath to Jonny Wilkinson at England, he's brilliant with us kids. Brian's only a little bloke but he's got the energy of 10 men. And because he's a northerner, not your typical rugger man from the home counties, I instantly warm to him.

Brian is always trying to get us to think for ourselves, because he won't be on the field once the game starts. He sets up defences that seem impossible to break down, just to see what we'll come up with. One time, I say to my mate Dom Waldouck, 'I'm going to do a switch with you, carry on drifting across their defence, before bouncing the ball between my legs. So be ready.' Brian blows his whistle, we do what I said we were going to do, the defenders all stop, Dom goes through the gaping hole I've created and scores. I'm not being flash, or messing about, I'm trying to solve Brian's seemingly impossible conundrum. Brian loves it.

Brian is about seeing and feeling, creating an enabling environment, empowering us to be ourselves, rather than churning out mini versions of him. He has this old military saying: 'No battle plan survives contact with the enemy.' So instead of rigid game-plans, Brian comes up with ideas and concepts and lets us play around with them. We don't always get things right, but all that experimenting is making our minds more elastic. And it suits me down to the ground, because I've never had much structure in my life.

Brian makes me feel special, but it's not as if he's constantly showering me with love and letting me have everything my own way. Him and his team are trying to make us think like professionals, which means eating the right things, staying hydrated, going to bed early and spending plenty of time in the gym. One day, I'm invited to Twickenham, for a session with Jonny Wilkinson and his kicking coach Dave Alred. I like Jonny, he's kind and generous. And every time he kicks the ball to me, I don't have to move. That, Dave tells me, is down to hard work, not magic.

My biggest fall-out with Brian happens when I get my mate Dom to piss in a cup before a hydration test (it was six in the morning, and I didn't need to pee). When the results come back, they show my pee is chemically identical to Dom's, which is a one in a billion chance. Brian gives me a proper bollocking and sends me home.

But mostly Brian's training camps are amazing experiences. I enjoy them so much I've stopped going to Tobago for my summer holidays, which means I only hear from Dad on the phone every now and again.

Wasps' academy is full of talent, including quite a few kids I've played against. Guys like Dom, who my dad taught to swim and played for Rosslyn Park's arch-rivals Richmond, Tom Rees and James Haskell. Haskell is this massive bloke who's never out of the gym and doesn't stop talking. When he's off on one, the boys will be looking at each other as if to say, 'Where the hell did this nutcase come from?' I think he'll go a long way.

Shaun Edwards, who's the defence coach for the first team and a rugby league legend, won tons with Wigan but hasn't been in union long. He's this gruff northerner with a mad bastard resting face, teeth missing, and a nose bent halfway across his head, so a lot of the lads are shit scared of him. Like a lot of them, I went to a private school. The difference is, I've spent a lot of time around working-class people, so Shaun doesn't really faze me.

I walk into the gym one day and Shaun is punching the heavy bag in his Y-fronts. He always does that, it's not like anyone is going to take the piss out of him. He's really getting into it, letting his hands fly, but I walk up to him and say, 'Shaun, why have you got a tattoo of your own face on your arm?' Shaun stops punching and replies, 'It's not a tattoo of me, it's me brother.'

Shaun tells me his brother recently died in a car crash and that it's devastated the family. He's this supposedly scary bloke, but here he is sharing his vulnerabilities with a 16-year-old kid he barely knows.

Suddenly, Shaun says, 'Right, can you hold these pads for me?' I stand in front of him, with the pads shoulder width apart, and he starts getting agitated – 'No, no, no! Tight to ya face! Tighter! Tighter!' I do as I'm told and he starts hammering away at the pads, growling every time he lands. I catch the odd stray punch on the ear, which stings a bit, but I don't mind. It's a privilege.

On Saturday mornings, I train with Shaun on my own. We'll be out there for hours, working on the intricacies of the sport – tempo, timing, speed of ball, stuff most 16-year-olds aren't learning. And when we're doing bits and pieces in the gym, he tells funny stories about fights he's had, on and off the field; his Catholic faith, which is so important to him; and his playing career: child prodigy, captain of England schoolboys in league and union (which I can't get my head around), the pressure of signing for the mighty Wigan on his 17th birthday.

Shaun's dad was a strict disciplinarian, and the only person whose opinion ever mattered to him. Meanwhile, Wigan was a world-class sporting environment light years ahead of anything in union. Make no mistake, Shaun knows more than pretty much anyone about sporting perfection.

* * *

Me and Dom start training with the first team when we're only 16. We rock up in our school uniform, hang our blazers and ties on pegs, before going out and cutting the old boys up, which we find hilarious. In secret.

Most of the lads are welcoming, but one or two seem irritated by our presence. Tim Payne doesn't stop giving me grief. He's a prop, so it's not like I'm going to take his place. Maybe he's fuming because I'm this kid who's getting special treatment, running about like I don't have a care in the world.

Me and Dom are playing against the first team and Shaun's trying out his famous blitz defence, which is the big innovation he brought over from league. We're up against all these England players – Lawrence Dallaglio, Matt Dawson, Joe Worsley, Phil Vickery, Simon Shaw, Alex King, Paul Sackey – but it doesn't take me long to work out that Shaun's blitz defence can be unlocked.

I'm standing there thinking, *Those defenders are normally up so quick that the ball-carrier either takes the tackle or panics and throws a dodgy pass, meaning the next man gets nailed. But maybe if I slow my feet down and skip outside, the defender will jam in on me, creating separation from the next defender.* So I say to Dom, 'Follow my body language. I'm gonna skip outside, before straightening and playing it short to you.'

Sure enough, it works, and we cut through quite a few times. Shaun must be loving it, because all those one-on-one sessions are bearing fruit – and he knows he's about to get his hands on me full-time.

A few weeks after I turn 17, the head coach Warren Gatland tells me I'm playing for the first team at the weekend, albeit starting on the bench. I'm dumbstruck, but excited and ready to face whatever happens.

It's a domestic cup game against Bristol in their backyard and nobody seems too worried about it. The coach ride down there is the first time I've spoken to our captain Lawrence Dallaglio, although I did hold a door open for him once. I'm looking forward to his pre-match speech because I've heard they give you goosebumps and make the hairs on the back of your neck stand on end. But there's not much big chat on this occasion, it's all quite low-key. I'm assuming he saves the Churchill stuff for games like the World Cup final.

If it was a close game, Gats wouldn't put me on. But we're hammering them, so I play the last five minutes. Just after taking up my position at fly-half, someone shouts, 'Munster!', and I think, *What does that mean?* One of the forwards gets the ball, two or three more big lads go with him, and I blindly follow. The ball pops out the back, the scrum-half passes it to me and I boot it cross-field to Josh Lewsey on the wing. That's my first act in proper grown-up rugby.

The remaining few minutes are a blur. I don't feel out of place, although everything is much faster and more physical. And because no-one's told me what I'm supposed to be doing, I'm having to freestyle. But that's fine by me.

After the match, I can't stop thinking about something Matt Dawson said to me: 'Danny, you've got all the talent in the world, but you've got to play the game,' by which he meant my general demeanor, rather than the way I play rugby. Matt's a World Cup winner and is just being nice and sharing some of his wisdom, but it doesn't sit right with me.

Play the game? I'm playing rugby how I think it should be played, isn't that enough? Does he mean I have to be fake, say things I don't believe, do things that aren't me? I don't want to do that. If I feel something, I feel something. I'm true to myself and that's the way it's always going to be.

5

THE ORPHANAGE

At the Under-19 World Cup in South Africa, I smash my head on the ground in the semi-final against the hosts. Stretchered off, apparently. Next thing I know, I'm in hospital phoning Mum, asking her to come and see me.

'Danny,' she says, 'I'm in England.'

'Mum,' I reply, 'stop mucking about. I know you're next door.'

I'm out of it for hours. When I come round, they tell me I've got a bleed on the brain. 'Did we win?' I ask the doctor. 'Sorry, no,' he replies.

Whenever I try to exercise, I feel light-headed. This goes on for six months, during which time I do pretty much nothing, apart from riding an exercise bike. One day, someone tells me about an interview Gats has done, in which he says I could be a bigger star than Jonny Wilkinson. I love Jonny – everyone loves Jonny, he's the golden boy who kicked the goal that won the World Cup for England – so I'm taken aback. But I'm chuffed as well.

The following year, spring 2006, I'm playing against South Africa in the Under-19s World Cup again, this time in Dubai. I put my head in the wrong place making a tackle, and even though I'm now wearing a scrum hat, I get knocked out again. At least this time we win the game.

I'm only out for three weeks this time, and no-one seems concerned about all these whacks on the head. 'Just make sure you keep wearing a scrum hat, you'll be alright.' And once I've finished my exams and packed up school, I have a bit of a break before I join up with Wasps' academy full-time.

Adam Thompstone has landed a full-time gig with London Irish, but they've let Nev go. All Nev ever wanted to do was play rugby for a living, so he's really upset. Now he's off to university, like most other kids. Meanwhile, I'm off to play professional rugby while Mum wants me to go to university.

Some of my team-mates look more like bodybuilders than rugby players, and they're still only teenagers. They don't move easily, it all seems like an effort, a little bit stressful, like they need a squirt of WD-40.

They've had me lifting weights since I was 15, and recently we've been in the gym three times a day, lifting heavy for as long as possible. That's on top of the actual rugby.

I understand the approach because a focus on physicality is a big part of Wasps' success. And I enjoy the animalistic aspect of shifting weights, and demonstrating I can lift more than some of the forwards. But sometimes I feel stiff just walking about, because of the extra muscle. And I've lost some of my sharpness. I'm still gliding past and ghosting through defenders, but I don't have the same change of speed, like my hero Christian Cullen. That won't do.

I tell Ian McGeechan, our director of rugby, I want to train with Margot Wells, who's a sprint coach I've been seeing for six months already (leave school, catch the 4.30 train to Guildford, arrive at 5.30, train with Margot until 7, get home at 8.30). Geech replies, 'Take the time off, Danny. It's going to be a gruelling pre-season and you've got a long career ahead of you.'

Geech coached the Lions to victory in South Africa a few years ago, but I don't take any notice of him. Instead, I train with Margot Monday to Saturday for the next six weeks. When we do the first speed test of pre-season, I'm faster than I've ever been. I even beat Josh Lewsey and Paul Sackey who's meant to be the quickest in the squad.

Geech takes me aside and says, 'Have you been seeing Margot?'

'Yep,' I reply.

Geech gives me a little smile and says, 'Well, you can keep on seeing her. Just make sure you keep everyone up to date.'

The problem is, Wasps' conditioners want me to stick to their programme, they don't like me doing my own thing. I tell them I'm doing what Margot wants me to do. They don't look happy, but they're not going to change my mind.

Margot's made me think about weights in a whole different way. I still do half of Wasps' programme, but don't lift weights to the point of exhaustion – speed and power is always the emphasis. The coaches get it, because they see

Margot's way is benefiting me. But I get the impression the conditioners think I'm being disruptive. The way I see it, I'm not being different for the sake of being different, I'm just doing whatever I need to do to improve.

If Dad was around, I'd discuss it with him. But he's not. As for Mum, she's always telling me how hard she's worked to get me where I am, so telling her I've gone rogue wouldn't go down too well. I'm already my own man at 17.

After Gats leaves to take charge of Wales, Shaun takes over as head coach. Shaun calls us a team full of reprobates, or an orphanage. That chimes with me, because I've always felt a bit like an orphan.

It's a very professional environment, and Shaun doesn't accept half-hearted, but it's not what you'd call a typical rugby team. Haskell went to one of the most exclusive schools in the country but arrived at Wasps with a big black mark against his name (something to do with filming his mate having sex, although he pleads not guilty). Luckily for Hask, rascals are embraced at Wasps, considered to one of the family, part of the furniture. The fact he trains like a maniac obviously helps.

Like Hask, Lawrence went to a top private school. But, like me, he has working-class roots. He's also been through a lot of adversity, what with his sister dying in the *Marchioness* boat disaster and him being accused by the papers of dealing drugs, which meant he lost the England captaincy. I think that's the reason Lawrence and Shaun are so close, because they've shared a lot of heartache.

Of the old boys, Phil Vickery and Simon Shaw have taken me under their wings. Phil's the son of a Cornish dairy farmer and hard as nails, but he's gentle enough with me. Shawsey's a bit harsher but seems to be softening up a bit. I'm still not sure what to make of Tim Payne. He'll look at me like I'm a piece of shit and I'll think, *Why does this guy hate me so much?*

I find Payney fascinating. Here's this miserable old prop, who drinks ludicrous amounts of alcohol and looks more like a trucker than an athlete, but he's phenomenal in fitness tests. And when he plays, he never gets tired. How is he able to do that? That's what I mean about this Wasps team, everyone has hidden depths. And Payney has more hidden depths than most.

Alex King is the first team fly-half and he's a club legend who knows his business inside out. But the other day, Shaun said to me, 'Everything Alex can do, you can learn. But some of the things you can do, Alex can't.' I love that, it makes me feel special. It also explains why Alex is friendly enough but definitely holding things back. He knows, like Shaun knows, that I'll be taking his place soon enough, but he's not ready to give up all his secrets yet.

Shaun sees my future at 10, and trains me as such. But because of the speed work I've been doing with Margot, I'm slick enough to play full-back. Shaun just wants to fit me in the team, because he thinks I'll make stuff happen. I've never played 15 before, so Shaun gives me three basic pointers: run hard, pass early, the rest you'll just know. *Okay, Shaun, if you say so.*

People think Shaun is just a great technical coach, but he's also a psychological genius. I'll give you an example. One morning, I'm walking down the corridor, Shaun's walking towards me and I'm trying to catch his eye. Usually he'll say, 'Alright, Danny? Have a good weekend? See you out there.' But this time he's got a face like thunder and blanks me. So now I'm thinking, *I don't want to piss him off today, better be bang on it.* And when I get on the field, I train the house down.

With Shaun, like with Brian Ashton, you get the sense it's all from the heart, not from books. They're people coaches, emotionally intelligent. As a player, Shaun was known for being unbelievably driven, and he's got this uncanny ability to breathe that attitude into the players he coaches. Half an hour with Shaun and you want to be the best it's possible to be.

Shaun picks me on the bench for the game against Bath, my Premiership debut. I come on with 20 minutes to go and score my first try as a professional, an interception from 70-odd metres out. That must have shocked a few fans – they thought they were getting a ball-playing fly-half, not an out-and-out speedster. Even better, we batter Bath 47–18.

When our regular full-back Mark van Gisbergen goes on his honeymoon, I get my first Premiership start against Worcester, score our only try and win man of the match. I also start in our win against Perpignan in the Heineken Cup, but when Mark returns, he wins his place back.

There's a bit of toing and froing, but Shaun picks me for the Heineken Cup quarter-final against Leinster and the papers are talking about a changing of the guard. Because it's not just me who's impressing, Dom's also tearing up trees in the centres and Hask and Tom Rees are back-row regulars. There's a real excitement around the place, a feeling that Wasps' future is going to be bright.

Because the Leinster game is a big 'un, I get a better look at what Lawrence is all about as a captain. When he speaks in the changing room before kick-off, you can tell he's lived a life outside of rugby. It's all there – anger, desperation, frustration and lots more besides. Lawrence is all in, which makes me want to follow him.

All the same, I've got no idea why Joe Worsley's banging his head against the wall. I've spoken to Joe, he's an intelligent, articulate guy, so now I'm looking at him thinking, *What's happened to you? How is that helping?* Everyone else seems to think it's perfectly normal.

Leinster are missing Brian O'Driscoll, who can play a bit, but their backline is still full of seasoned internationals – Gordon D'Arcy, Denis Hickie, Shane Horgan and Girvan Dempsey, plus Argentina's Felipe Contepomi at fly-half. So I can't understand why they're playing like idiots. Elbows in my face, knees in my ribs, a load of dumb faux hardman shit. Josh Lewsey even has to fight one of them for me. After another shoeing in a ruck, I'm thinking, *This ain't professional rugby. And you're grown men! Go and improve your skills so you don't feel the need to bully a 19-year-old kid.*

If Leinster's tactics had worked, fair enough I suppose. But we stuff them, scoring four tries to one, two of them while our skipper is in the sin-bin. Whenever I get the ball,

I do what Shaun told me: pass early to the winger or run as hard as possible. On this particular day, 'the rest' doesn't come into it. When I score my try, I lose my shit and scream in their faces.

Shaun's right, you get a good view of things from full-back. And that day, Kingy gives an object lesson in how to lead by example and run a game from fly-half. Nothing fancy, just shrewd. More about logistics than tricks, making sure everything is done just right. Meanwhile, Lawrence manages to combine being a scarily ferocious rugby player with faultless diplomacy. One second he's smoking someone in a tackle, the next he's having a polite chat with the ref – Yes, sir, no, sir – like butter wouldn't melt in his mouth.

I feel a bit bad for Mark van Gisbergen, because he's a Wasps stalwart and an awesome bloke. I can tell he's a bit down that I've taken his place, but he's still giving me loads of advice on full-back play. There's no way Shaun would put up with any moping anyway. If someone takes your place you knuckle down and try to win it back, or you'll get binned in a heartbeat.

Shaun's big on excellence and discipline, but he also wants people to be themselves. He gives players rope, as long as they put the work in during training and do the business at the weekend. Take Paul Sackey. We'll be in the middle of a team run and hear some old-school garage coming from the car park. Cue stifled laughter. Then we'll see Sacks strolling across the field. And when I say strolling, I mean *stro-llll-ing*. When he finally catches up with us, he'll say, in his South London drawl, 'Sorry boys, but I'll be on it tomorrow. You know that for a fact.' And because he's almost always true to his word, Shaun lets it slide.

Then there's Josh Lewsey. What a character he is. I think he likes me, but sometimes he looks at me like I'm some weird creature that's washed up on the beach. And he trains nothing like he plays on a Saturday.

Josh is still really quick, seriously strong, great under the high ball, with decent skills. But in training, he thinks he's David Campese. He'll do all this flash stuff he'd never do in a match – stepping off his wing, throwing Hollywood passes – and almost none of it comes off. Team-mates are throwing their arms in the air, puffing out their cheeks, but Shaun knows Josh will go back to basics at the weekend and do his job properly.

Shaun even gives himself rope. He'll wear a suit with a bomber jacket and a pair of Puma Kings. Or a suit jacket, tracksuit bottoms and smart shoes. There are always a couple of bits wrong. Sometimes, I think he's doing it deliberately, to mess with our heads. Then I think he's not as calculating as that. Thinking about it, it's the opposite of wrong, he's doing what feels right.

When you let everyone be individuals, there's no rigid hierarchy, all those traditional dividing lines become blurred. The pups aren't intimidated by the old beasts and the old beasts are energised by the pups. That's why there's a unity that runs through this team, from top to bottom. Even the lads who spend most of their time on the bench are working their nuts off, because they're terrified of being jettisoned from such an accepting environment.

6

I'M GONNA DO ME

While Lawrence is doing his Churchill thing before the Heineken Cup semi-final against Northampton, Sacks is slunk in the corner, muttering, 'It'll be alright, Dan. Just give me the ball and I'll do what I want. All. Day. Long.'

'Okay,' I reply, 'cool.'

Kingy's got a knock, so I'm starting at 10, up against Carlos Spencer – 40-odd caps for New Zealand and a whizz at unlocking defences. I see what he's all about just a few minutes in, when he lobs an overhead pass to his former All Black mate Bruce Reihana, who goes over in the corner.

Twenty minutes in and we're 13–0 down. For the second week running, I blow a try by touching the ball down on the in-goal whitewash. Sloppy, not something Kingy would do. No matter. For the rest of the game, our pack grinds them into dust. Whenever I give Sacks the ball, he does what he wants, like he said he would. He ends up scoring two and we march on to the final.

Our Heineken Cup final opponents Leicester have already completed a domestic league and cup double. But while they've been slogging their guts out for the whole of May, we've been fine-tuning.

A week before we meet at Twickenham, Leicester demolish Gloucester in the Premiership final. Their Samoan winger Alesana Tuilagi, who's built like a cement mixer but can shift like a Ferrari, tramples all over them and scores two tries. It's like watching a cartoon, defenders flying everywhere. So on the Monday, Shaun says to me, 'Let's keep working on that Cumberland roll ...'

When big wingers like Tuilagi make line breaks, it's bloody difficult to chop them down at the legs. So Shaun comes up with the idea of knocking their hand-off out of the way, hitting up top as hard as you can and using their body weight to flip them, like a judo roll. No idea where Shaun got the Cumberland bit from.

They've patched Kingy up, so I'm starting at 15. Fine by me. This time, Lawrence reduces some people to tears before kick-off. That's the thing about Lawrence, he knows exactly what to do and say at the right time (apart from that time he crushed a plastic cup, while roaring, 'LET'S FUCKING DO IT!', which everyone laughed at). No point going full throttle before a dead league match against whoever's bottom of the table, because you won't feel the difference when it's the big occasion.

Leicester are never really in it. In the first half, we score off a couple of trick line-out plays, which the forwards have been practising for weeks. Kingy does the rest with his boot and we're almost home and dry. With about five minutes to go, they lob the ball over the top, Tuilagi receives it out wide and heads straight for me. Now I know what a bullfighter feels like. When he's close enough, I knock his hand-off out of the way, hit him up top as hard as I can and flip him into touch. Just like I've been working on with Shaun.

After the game, Shaun strolls into the dinner wearing trainers with his suit. I say to him, 'Shaun, why the trainers?' He replies, 'Danny, let me tell you something. If you ever get into a fight and you've got slippery shoes on, like a fancy pair of winkle-pickers, you've got no leverage. Happened to me once. I were exchanging blows outside the pub, slipped, and got me head kicked in.'

I'm thinking, *I know some of Leicester's players are bad losers, but still.*

As I'm leaving, I can hear Shaun holding court. 'How about when Tuilagi was running at Danny,' he says. 'Cumberland rolls him! Bosh, into touch, fuckin' great!'

Brian's now England head coach and he's picked me for his first World Cup training squad. He probably saw me cut up New Zealand Maori playing for England's second string. I felt on one that day, lit the place up.

When I turn up, it's all these blokes who won the World Cup four years ago. The Wasps lads, obviously, but also Jonny Wilkinson, Mike Catt, Mike Tindall and Jason Robinson, all household names. I have to admit, it's pretty mind-blowing – I was still at school last year. But you'd be a mug to just stand around gawking and soaking up the atmosphere, so I talk to Jonny about fly-half play and to Jason about footwork, and they're only too happy to help.

Brian takes us on a Special Forces training camp, which is a bloody nightmare. We think we're off to Portugal until someone shouts, 'We're not going towards the airport, lads!' A couple of hours later, I'm running through a lake with a canoe on my back, thinking, *Why the fuck am I doing this?*

I can tell some of the senior players have got the hump, big time. Some drop out early, saying they need to protect long-term injuries. Some drop out early simply because they think it's a load of old bollocks.

Brian likes me, but the chances of him taking me to France are slim to none. I make it through the first cull, which means I'm on the bench for the warm-up game against France. But even though it doesn't go to plan, Brian doesn't put me on. As the clock ticks down at Twickenham, they shove a camera in my face and show me on the big screen, looking miserable. I just wish Brian had given me the opportunity to prove myself.

When I first hear that England's players turned against Brian at the World Cup, I can't understand it. Now players are saying England reaching the final – and coming within a whisker of winning it – had nothing to do with him. Lawrence says there was no leadership and that it was like playing in a pub team.

Having given it more thought, it makes a lot of sense. Brian has an idea of how the game should be played but he doesn't believe in game-plans. He's not prescriptive, he's about freedom of choice, players taking responsibility. That was an ageing England squad, with a lot of strong personalities, so imagine being that type of innovative, imaginative coach in a room full of rugby players who've been around the block a few times. You're trying to create an environment in which they work things out for themselves and they're thinking, *Can't you just tell us what to do? Then we'll go and do it.*

Ironically, because Brian had the nous to take a step back, the players ended up doing it their way, which is what Brian wanted them to do in the first place. By being humble, Brian got what he wanted, as did the players. The problem was, the players thought they'd done it all despite him.

Kingy's gone to play for Clermont in France. I don't know if he thought his place in the team was under threat, but the move makes sense for both of us. Kingy's in his thirties, out of the England reckoning and can make a nice few quid before retiring. During pre-season, Shaun says to me, 'Now you're the man.'

I'm a proper rugby geek, constantly honing my craft. Because rugby is a craft, at least to me. When I hold a rugby ball, I imagine it must feel like an instrument feels in the hands of a musician.

I spend hours working with Shaun on more high-brow stuff, like analysing the movement of defenders and how to make holes in defences. But we also talk a lot about simplifying my game. Shaun says that by doing most things simply, you'll have a better idea of when the big play is on. Instead of feeling forced, you'll feel compelled.

We get off to an iffy start to the 2007–08 season, winning only one of our first six games. But when the cavalry returns from World Cup duty in France, things begin to change. Shaun's given me permission to be me, but because I'm part of an unbelievable group of players, I'm not taking many risks. I don't need to when the team around me is functioning so well.

It helps that I've got Riki Flutey outside me at 12. What a great addition he is, such great skills and vision. He's also completely bonkers. When we play Llanelli in Wales, we share a room, and when the lights go out, he's snoring his head off within seconds of his head hitting the pillow. Half an hour goes by, still snoring. An hour goes by, still snoring. I don't feel like I can say anything because he's a senior player. *As long as he's getting a good night's sleep*, I think, *that's all that matters*. But after an hour and a half, I finally snap.

'For fuck's sake, Riki, stop fucking snoring!'

Riki opens one eye and replies, 'Gotcha, bro! I wasn't even sleeping!'

'Please don't tell me you've been fake snoring for an hour and a half?'

'Yeah, bro!'

When I do something most fly-halves don't do, I don't consider it a risk. I'm just trying to do what I think is best for the team in that moment, like I did at school. And if it doesn't come off, I won't stop doing it, I'll just do it better next time.

I've heard people say, 'Cipriani will win you games, but he'll also lose you the odd one.' That's a great place to be at my age, because by learning from those mistakes, the more I'll improve, and the more amazing things I'll do.

We're into November and I feel untouchable. I sense teams fear me, that I've got them in a tizz even before we walk onto the pitch. 'What's this kid gonna do? How are we gonna neutralise him?'

When we beat Munster in the Heineken Cup, I go head-to-head with Ireland veteran Ronan O'Gara and more than match him. When the final whistle goes, the camera pans to me and I throw my scrum hat in the air, like a student at his graduation.

One day after training, Geech says to me, 'Danny, you've got to slow down a bit because the other lads aren't at your level.' I think, *What the hell? Why would you want me to slow down? It's your job to make them see what I'm seeing. We're playing professional sport, here, not tag in the playground.*

Imagine an LA Lakers coach saying to Kobe Bryant, 'Stop doing all that creative stuff because your team-mates aren't good enough to keep up.' Madness. Wouldn't happen, because it's a self-defeating attitude. An NBA coach would take the time to work out what his key player is doing, communicate that to the rest of his players and get them suitably upskilled.

Thank God Shaun's different. If I overdo things in a game, he lets me know, maybe by ignoring me before training. But he never comes down hard on me for expressing myself. He wants me to be the best player I can be, and the only way that's going to happen is if I try things, make mistakes and learn from them.

Before some games, I know I'm not going to have to bring the physical stuff, because we're going to score more tries than them. People in rugby hate that attitude. You get players and coaches constantly screaming, 'YOU'VE GOT TO PUT YOUR BODY ON THE LINE!' Shaun will give me a hard time if I miss a tackle, don't worry about that, but he knows I can do things with the ball my team-mates can't, so he gives me more leeway, even though that goes against one of the cardinal rules of rugby, which is that everyone should be treated the same. That kind of attitude leaves little room for individuals to do their thing.

Before a big game, like the Heineken Cup final, Shaun will put an arm around me and say, 'Danny, I need you today physically.' And I'll reply, 'Of course.' End of discussion. Because he treats me with respect, and I'm emotionally invested, he knows I'll run through brick walls for him.

SHAUN EDWARDS

I'd been hearing about Danny from when he was 16 or 17, that we'd soon have our hands on this kid who was destined to be a superstar of the future.

When he started training with the first team, everybody could see he was special. We had some great players, World Cup winners, people who'd been playing at the highest level for years, but they all welcomed Danny with open arms. Danny wasn't intimidated by them, and he wasn't intimidated by me. He had no reason to be, because I wanted to help him.

When Danny says I was one of the only coaches who saw him for who he truly was, that didn't happen by accident. Mine and Danny's stories are similar. I signed for Wigan in a blaze of publicity in 1983, on my 17th birthday. It was live on TV, watched by millions. So I understood more than most the intense scrutiny Danny was under, that weight of expectation.

We'd do one-on-one sessions together, talking about tactics, attacking patterns, different styles of passing. And he was a joy to work with. He had a great skillset, but was also quick, so I suggested to Ian McGeechan that we try him at full-back. That's where I played when I first joined Wigan, before switching to stand-off, and I know you can learn a lot from back there.

When I was a schoolboy at St John Fisher in Wigan, we had a coach called Mr McLeod, whose methods were miles ahead of what anybody else was doing. Mr McLeod was big on his tactics and his fitness, but he also wanted people to express their individuality on the field. It wasn't much different when I signed for Wigan, and I took that approach into my coaching career.

You've got to have a set of rules, like turning up on time and being polite, but I've never subscribed to this notion that everything has to be regimented and everybody has to fit in. You've got to give your all in training, and when you get on the pitch on game day, you have to stick to a structure. But you have to have individualism within that structure, and when you're not training or playing, you should be able to do what you want, within reason.

Mr McLeod was one of those characters who'd give you a little more rope once you'd earned his respect, and Danny earned my respect very quickly. As well as the work he did with me, he trained on his own and paid for extra sprint coaching. But Danny did occasionally test my patience.

I remember him turning up late for a training session, running on to the pitch and me barking at him, 'What do you think you're doing?' He replied, 'Sorry I'm late.' And I said, 'No you're not. Go and stand over there. You can watch, but you're not getting involved.' I can see him now, standing on the touchline, looking forlorn and slightly angry. What I didn't realise was that Danny was travelling miles to training, and not being a Londoner, I didn't realise how bad the traffic could be.

You've got to make allowances for different kinds of people in a team environment. For example, with some players, you've got to deliver criticism more gently. But I could be quite abrupt, even harsh, with Danny and he'd take it in the spirit it was intended. There certainly wouldn't be any tantrums or sulking. Maybe that's because we're similar personalities, and he's quite abrupt as well.

When people ask for my favourite moment coaching Danny Cipriani, they expect me to talk about an amazing pass he made or try he scored. But it's definitely that tackle he made on Alesana Tuilagi in the Heineken Cup final. We'd been practising that tackle for three or four months, so to see Danny execute it on a stage like that was magic: shoulder lined up perfectly, the flip into touch, everything we'd spent so long working on. That was special.

Then there was the time I promised Danny I'd buy him a bottle of champagne if he forced a turnover during the course of the season. It took him a while, but when he finally did, he celebrated like he'd scored the winning try.

Some people thought Danny was frail defensively, but his tackling was rarely an issue for me. I'd have him defending in the 13 channel, not because I was trying to hide him, but because it suited him down to the ground. He was a very good side-on tackler, and quicker than most 10s, so didn't get isolated. On top of that, I knew, from playing stand-off in rugby league, that if you're forced into making a lot of tackles, you get tired out and become less effective in attack. But by defending at 13, Danny was cutting down on his tackles, staying fresher and sharper, and being more dangerous with ball in hand.

The greatest testament to Danny's dedication, determination and resilience is how he came back from that horrific injury he suffered in 2008. I'm not sure people know how bad that injury was – it was a potential career-ender – but Danny was back well ahead of schedule and became a better player. He'd lost some of his pace, but his organisational skills and spatial awareness improved, and he became a more dominant leader.

Danny is very demanding, but fly-halves should be. He's the leader of the attack, and a big part of his job is to get the best out of everybody around him. When you're the guy barking orders, you can't be worrying about people getting offended and not liking you. The only thing anyone should be worrying about is winning. I know that, because I spent a lot of time barking orders at Wigan. That sometimes made me unpopular, but we won a hell of a lot.

There's not much to say about Danny's England career. He was competing with Owen Farrell for the best part of a decade, and Owen played for a dominant Saracens team. And when you play for a dominant team, you've got more chance of playing for England. Simple as that. Plus, Owen is a great player.

But for Danny to do what he did at Sale, Wasps second time around and Gloucester, he had to be a force of nature, because they all improved after his arrival, and they all played more exciting rugby.

If he asked, I'd advise him to get his coaching badges and pass all that knowledge on to youngsters. English rugby would certainly be better for it. But whatever he decides to do, I hope our friendship will continue throughout our lives. He knows I'm always on the end of the phone for him, and I'm sure he'd say the same about me.

7

ON DAYS LIKE THESE

There's a story in the *News of the World* about me two-timing a pop star. Didn't see that coming. And it gets worse.

I met this pop star at some do in London. It was a brief encounter, and her mum was her manager and chaperone, like something from Victorian times. So after chatting with her for a while, I thought that was the end of it. But then I read that me and this girl were an item. Then a few days later, a story came out that I'd been unfaithful to her – 'A LOVE RAT!' – with some reality TV character.

The thing is, I did sleep with this reality TV character, but most of the stuff she's told the *News of the World* is bullshit. She claims that while we were having sex, I kept saying how good we'd look on the beach together. It gets much worse: now it's come out that she used to be a bloke called Darren.

I walk into the changing room on Monday morning and there are copies of the *News of the World* spread all over the place. Hask looks happier than when we won the Heineken Cup, a look of pure glee on his face. Even

Tim Payne's smiling. The flak's flying thick and fast, but I decide to plough straight through the middle of it. I say to Hask, 'You can laugh all you like, but she's still fitter than your missus.' That kills them stone dead, because it's true.

Of course it's humiliating, but you've got two choices in a situation like that: face it or run from it. If you choose to run, it will be chasing you forever. Face it, and appear not to feel humiliated, and eventually you'll be free from it.

The changing room banter can be brutal, I can't be doing with a lot of it. Fair enough, have a bit of a joke, but some of it is way over the top, bordering on bullying. Some lads just don't feel comfortable with that level of piss-taking. Maybe they're not sharp enough, maybe they're just kind, gentle souls who happen to play a tough sport. Problem is, there's a herd mentality in rugby, and if you don't join in, you're tagged as an outsider, not to be trusted.

The same goes for nights on the piss. I'll sometimes go out with the lads but I'm not much of a boozer. I barely touched a drop the night we won the Heineken Cup. How can anyone like beer? It tastes rank. I'm convinced people only drink it because they think it makes them more manly.

My team-mates probably think I'm boring, but I couldn't care less. And because I'm fly-half for the first team, they let it slide. But fringe players are cast adrift if they'd rather have a quiet night in than down lager from some prop's manky old shoe. People in rugby are always going on about what an inclusive sport it is, how accepting it is of everyone. But it's not. If you don't stay in the herd, it can be a bit of a nightmare.

The same week the Darren story comes out, I play against Jonny Wilkinson for the first time. At the front end of the papers they're laughing at me, at the back end they're hyping me up as Jonny's successor as England's number 10.

We beat Jonny's Newcastle quite handily, but we've got a far better squad than them, so it proves nothing. It's only after our game against Clermont in the Heineken Cup that people really start talking me up.

Clermont are a great side, with my old team-mate Kingy at fly-half, but we're sensational in the first 40 minutes and I make four or five clean line breaks. I get a bit carried away in the second half, trying to force things instead of doing what's right in the moment, which lets them back in the game. But we hang on for the win and Shaun is happy enough.

Brian names me in his Six Nations squad, along with Jonny. I say all the right things to the press, and I mean every word. I'm on a mission to play for England, have been since I was 15, and I genuinely love Jonny, he's the greatest 10 this country's ever seen. But it's a media dream, a 20-year-old who's playing out of his skin against a legend who's hit a rough patch.

Journalists seem fascinated by the fact my mum's a cab driver. It's a bit patronising – 'READ ALL ABOUT IT! WORKING-CLASS RUGBY PLAYER!' – but I understand they've got to have angles. I tell journalists I owe everything to my mum and how much I love her, but only because I've seen other athletes do it.

Mum has worked hard and ducked and dived to send me to the schools she sent me to, but she doesn't have much of a maternal instinct. It's a hard, gristly love that's difficult to swallow.

Mum keeps a scrapbook of my rugby highlights, but she's never told me how happy or proud I make her. When I made my debut for Wasps, it was a case of, 'Well done, now on to the next thing.' When that kiss and tell story appeared in the *News of the World*, she told me how ashamed she was, without asking me for my side of the story.

Since I turned pro, it feels to me that it's all about money. 'How much are you earning? How much have you got in the bank?' It makes me feel uncomfortable and I hate it.

Meanwhile, Dad's started tapping me up. He'll call me, we'll be having a normal chat, and suddenly he'll ask if I can send him a few quid. He can never hold down a job, and it's always some other arsehole's fault. 'Dan,' he'll say, 'I'm struggling, I'm skint, I can't fend for myself.' It's my duty to help him, because I'm his son. But sometimes I'll hang up and think, *Did he even want to speak to me, or was it all to do with the money?*

Brian picks me on the bench for England's Six Nations opener against Wales. I feel like I should be starting instead of Jonny, because I'm playing with such confidence. But I'm not put out, and I know I'll be ready when Brian finally picks me.

I'm immensely proud to be selected for England. But the pride of getting picked to play for your country doesn't stem from patriotism – doing it for the Red Rose, St George, the Queen and all that. The way I look at it, I just happened to be born in England, by a zillion to one chance. So my pride is more personal. It stems from reaching the pinnacle of my sport, pitting myself against the best, and hopefully being seen as the best. If an England team I'm part of can get people excited, that's obviously a bonus.

The fans at Twickenham aren't exactly brimming with pride after our first Six Nations game against Wales. How we lose I do not know. One minute we're tearing them to shreds, the next we're shipping points all over the pitch.

I replace Mike Tindall at centre with 25 minutes to go, just before Lee Byrne goes over to level the scores. My first touch in international rugby comes from a wild pass from Jonny, miles over my head. I somehow manage to reel it in but get smashed. A couple of minutes later, Iain Balshaw's attempted clearance is charged down, Mike Phillips scores and Wales have won at Twickenham for the first time in 20 years.

Jonny gets a rinsing in the papers. Some pundits reckon he's over the hill, a busted flush, and that I should replace him for our next game against Italy. That doesn't happen and we're terrible again. I come on for Jonny with 14 minutes to go and have an attempted chip and chase charged down, which leads to a try. We hang on for a narrow win, but no-one's impressed.

Before the game against France, I play for Wasps against Bath. Shaun's landed a second job as Wales defence coach, so Geech is in charge. He says to me in the changing room, 'Danny, let's be calm today, nothing too risky.' It's like a red rag to a bull. Early on, we're struggling to break Bath down, so I attempt the same chip and chase that went wrong against Italy. Only this time I recover the ball, go round Bath full-back Nick Abendanon and score.

That's me flexing. It's hard to tell talented young players to cut the fancy stuff because it might go wrong. That's a crazy way of coaching, a sure way of stunting growth and creativity. Geech could have said to me, 'Don't worry about last week, you'll work things out. If you think it's the right option, do it. And this time you'll do it right.'

Jonny being Jonny, he rolls back the years in Paris and leads us to victory. Everyone thinks he's the best thing since sliced bread all over again. I'm thinking, *Well, I'm not gonna be starting at 10 in this tournament*. But on the Monday of the Scotland game, Brian tells me he's starting me at full-back instead.

On Wednesday evening, I see my physio in Mayfair and don't get out of there until gone 11. I've promised a mate I'll get him tickets for the game and that I'll hand them over in a nearby nightclub. I forget the tickets but decide to pop in anyway, just to say hello. I'm in the club for 20 minutes, at most, before jumping in my car and driving home. I'm in bed just after midnight.

When I wake up on Thursday, I see I've got a missed call from Brian. Plus quite a few texts. The first one says, 'Danny, you're on the front page of the papers.' Apparently, there are photos of me leaving the nightclub and the tabloids have added two and two and got five, accidentally on purpose.

Brian tells me he's had to drop me. I explain I just popped in for 20 minutes and didn't touch a drop, but his decision is made. He tells me he's not going to hold it against me, that it won't affect future selection, and I accept it.

I've known him since I was 15, he's always been good to me, and I trust he'll be true to his word. But all the time I'm thinking, *There were four or five other England guys drinking red wine around the corner, how is this fair?*

I don't know if Brian has been pushed into it by those above him or made the call off his own bat. Maybe he felt he had to flex his authority after what happened at the World Cup. *I'm in charge now, don't you dare defy me.*

The RFU officially charges me with 'inappropriate behaviour', but Brian gets a pasting in the papers, with some pundits accusing him of overreacting. Clive Woodward sounds furious, and Shaun has one or two words to say about it. But all that really matters is I won't be playing in Edinburgh on Saturday.

When Mum finds out, she's angrier with me than Brian. I know she loves boasting about me when she's driving the cab, because people have told me. But now I've made headlines for the wrong reasons. One thing's for certain, she won't be putting this in her scrapbook. It's all a bit overwhelming because I haven't done anything wrong.

* * *

England are abysmal against Scotland and lose 15–9. The press coverage is brutal, and I feel sorry for Jonny because he's getting so much stick. After the France game, he was the second coming of Jonny. Now he's all washed up again. But I'm also thinking, *Surely they've got to give me a shot at 10?*

On Monday, Brian tells me I'm starting instead of Jonny for the final game against Ireland. I knew Brian was a stand-up guy. All the same, you'd think he might tell me to keep my head down. Instead, he says, 'How do you want the week to go?' That takes me back a bit because I'm still only 20. Then again, people are calling for his head, so he probably doesn't think he's got much to lose: *Chuck Danny the keys and let him do whatever he needs to do.*

You can't upskill players in a week, but you can sharpen their focus, help them understand their roles better and give them the confidence to perform. So I sit down with Brian and explain my principles, knowing full well they're the same as his: not sticking religiously to a script, doing what's needed in the moment, telling players to trust themselves and play with freedom.

Brian has me taking meetings and running training sessions. I tell the lads we're simplifying the system. I give the forwards a bit of stick for being lazy. Brian's asked me to run the team, and you can't be a shrinking violet when you're playing 10. I twice cut training short. When Brian asks why, I tell him we're ready.

Jonny's being the magnanimous character he is: he shakes my hand, tells me he's 100 per cent behind me and says nice things about me to journalists. Funny thing is, Leicester's Toby Flood is starting outside me at 12, but when he picks up a knock in training, Jonny fills in for the first two sessions. It's spooky how well we connect. We're different players – I'm more about feel while Jonny is more meticulous – but we complement each other nicely. On the Wednesday, Brian says to me, 'Fuck, I wish I'd picked Jonny at 12 ...'

I read some bits and bobs in the papers and writers are calling me 'the clown prince' and 'enfant terrible'. I think, *What the hell's this based on? The fact I popped into a nightclub for 20 minutes three days before a game?*

I can't help thinking of Dennis Rodman when he was at the Chicago Bulls. Rodman went on a 48-hour bender in Vegas in the middle of an NBA season, which obviously his coaches and team-mates weren't happy about. But they found a way to deal with it: Michael Jordan went and dragged him out of bed and they got on with things. Head coach Phil Jackson could have come down hard on Rodman and punished him, but that would have made him resentful and of no use to the team. As it was, Jackson took a softly, softly approach and the Bulls ended up winning another NBA title.

People in rugby are always going on about their sport being a game of certain values – never complain, speak nicely to the ref, no play-acting like footballers, all this stuff that apparently makes us morally superior – but where's the honesty in what happened to me? Brian knew I rarely drank alcohol, as did everyone in the squad, but somehow I've ended up with a reputation as a loose cannon. I love what Phil Jackson said about the Rodman situation: 'There are different rules for different players.'

I get why players want to be told exactly what to do before they run out at Twickenham. There are 82,000 people in the stadium, plus millions watching on TV, so having a rigid role within a rigid game-plan makes them feel safe.

But rugby is an unpredictable game, with many moving parts, so being rigid in movement and thought isn't helpful. Even though I'm well-prepared, I don't really know what I'm going to do in the moment, and I feel ready to react to whatever happens around me.

I was up all night, only because I was looking forward to the game so much, like a kid on Christmas Eve. Sitting in the changing room, I can't think of anywhere else I'd rather be. But some of the lads look like they're being sent off to war. There's so much tension and what feels to me like apprehension.

There are seven minutes on the clock, we're 10–0 down and Twickenham sounds like ... well, like it's hosting something dismal. It's only when I drive the Irish deep into their own half with a pinpoint kick, we win a penalty and I pop over my first points for England that the crowd shows signs of life.

We're halfway through the first half when Sacks gets the ball in broken play and brushes off a couple of defenders. There follows some nice handling from the big fellas, the ball comes out to me, I spin it wide to Jamie Noon, he draws his man and passes it back to Sacks, who goes over in the corner.

A few minutes later, I open up a hole with a bit of footwork and a show of the ball, Noon slices through the middle and is held up just short. But when Ireland infringe at the breakdown, I kick us into the lead. As I'm running off at half-time, I think, *What's all the fuss about? This feels like a school game.*

Ireland are missing their vaunted pairing of Brian O'Driscoll and Gordon D'Arcy in the centres and they're a bit of a mess after the break. Our pack is on top, I'm getting plenty of front-foot ball, seeing space all over the field, and my team-mates are completely in synch. Nothing fancy, just doing simple things well, like Shaun taught me.

On days like these, it's like being at the controls of a precision machine, with everything working perfectly. I'm playing right on the line, drawing out defenders, and whenever I see a hole, I put someone through it. Short pass, long pass, it's all coming off. Whenever I punt, it's an effortless swing of the leg and the sweetest of connections. I can't miss from the tee either – even when the ball topples over and the ref tells me to take the kick quickly, I still manage to slot the conversion despite slipping and falling backwards.

Now one from the training ground: Lesley Vainikolo, who's built like a bison, comes charging off his wing and creates the extra man, before Mathew Tait finishes things off. Jonny comes on at inside-centre with 30 minutes to go, sending the crowd mental, before Noon adds another try before the final whistle. Seven kicks from seven, eighteen points on debut, Twickenham rocking like it hasn't done in ages. I think it's gone okay.

I'm still wildly excited when a reporter sticks a mic under my nose. I go off on a bit of a ramble, and while congratulating the forwards on their performance, drop the F-bomb. I immediately apologise, but I'm sure there are still plenty of disgusted viewers, spluttering into their tea, calling me a foul-mouthed yob and vowing to fire off a stern letter of complaint to the BBC.

But take out the swear word and I'm just an exuberant kid giving his heart to his team-mates, when I might have made it all about myself. If people choose to ignore the praise I was sharing, it says more about them than it does about me. I've got every right to be emotional, I've just fulfilled my dream.

8

FAIR GAME

It's the day after the game against Ireland and the papers are all calling me the saviour of English rugby, or variations on that theme. Meanwhile, poor Jonny is yesterday's man. That's a bit much, Jonny's not even 30, and I reckon we'd make a great partnership, with me at fly-half and him at 12. But that's the media for you, no nuance. They're all frustrated Hollywood scriptwriters.

Just a week ago, journalists were saying English rugby has never been lower. Now they're talking about a golden generation. Whether we are or not, Brian won't be leading us. Six months after almost winning the World Cup, he's been sacked and replaced by Martin Johnson.

I'd ride and die for Brian, he's my kind of coach. He's true to himself and wants his players to be true to themselves as well. But that's probably why they ditched him. Maybe the RFU don't want a head coach who does things his own way, maybe they want someone who just *sounds* and *looks* right instead.

Some of those older players were set in their ways. They wanted their head coach to fit in with them, not the other way around. If you want to be told what to do, like a robot being programmed, and if you want to be in control, because it makes you feel safe, Brian's not really your man.

One England player calls Brian 'romantic' in the papers. I assume that's code for 'unrealistic'. If you're open-minded and humble, happy to cast off long-held ideas and work on changing the way you play the game, eventually Brian's ideas won't seem romantic, they'll seem like the natural way of doing things. But if you've only ever been taught to run straight lines and crash into defenders, Brian coming in and trying to get you to understand that the game can look different is going to rankle. You're being put in an uncomfortable place, having to face up to your own limitations, accept that you don't know rugby as well as you think you do. And learning new things is hard work.

If they had to get rid of Brian, I don't understand how Shaun hasn't replaced him, or at least been given a role in Johnno's coaching set-up.

Before Shaun got the Wales gig, he rounded up Wasps' England players, sat us down in a meeting room and told us the RFU had offered him a part-time job coaching the Saxons, England's second string. He said he was passionate about England, and wanted to coach them, but the Welsh job offered more career opportunities and meant more money. I said, 'I completely understand, Shaun, sounds like the RFU are taking the piss.'

Everyone at Wasps thought the RFU had lost their minds. As far as we were concerned, Shaun was the best coach in England by a country mile. He ticked every box:

a great technical coach, defence and attack; brilliant at improving youngsters and upskilling more experienced players; deep emotional intelligence and inspiring beyond belief; a proven winner; a patriot.

I guess Shaun, like Brian, just didn't *sound* or *look* right. He's not someone the RFU blazers could put in a corner and tell what to do. He's going to say whatever he wants and do things exactly how he wants to. Nothing bland, no bullshit, straight down the line. A one-off, not from a mould.

Maybe I'm wrong and the RFU honestly think Johnno will do a better job. Maybe they're just not very bright, because if they were, Johnno wouldn't be anywhere near the England job. Yes, he was captain when England won the World Cup, but he's never coached anyone. They assume that because he was a great leader on the field, he'll be a great leader on the touchline. How naïve is that? He was a big, tough lock who did his job extremely well. But what's his philosophy? Never mind, he *sounds* and *looks* like English rugby is supposed to – A MAN OF STATURE, WHO'LL MAKE US ROAR! – and that's what counts to the RFU.

At first I think I've got really bad cramp. Only when I look at my ankle do I realise it's pointing the wrong way and there's a bone coming through my sock. That's when the pain and fear kick in.

Someone sticks an oxygen mask over my face and I hear them say, 'Fuck, this is a bad one.' Someone else who looks quite scared says they're going to have to put my ankle back in on the field. Behind the mask I blurt out, 'Just fucking do it!' It's like a scene from an old war film. They snap my ankle back into place, I scream a blood-curdling scream, and that's the end of the pain.

I emerge from surgery and the doc tells me I've suffered a fracture-dislocation that has gone through both the fibula and the tibia. Oh, and that I might never play rugby again. What do you say to that? Just a few hours ago I was playing in a Premiership semi-final, having just been named young player of the year. This was meant to be just the beginning of my time as England's number 10. And now I'm being told it's all gone up in smoke.

My physio Kevin Lidlow, who I've been seeing since I was 17, watched the surgery, and he's not listening to what the doctor is saying. I trust Kevin to tell me the truth, good or bad, and when he says it's gone well and he'll be able to get me back on the field – as long as I attack my rehab with the same mentality I've attacked everything else so far in my career – I believe him.

I'm laid up in bed with my leg elevated for the next two weeks. The only time I'm on my feet is when I need the toilet, and even then I do it in a pot. Luckily, I've got two good girlfriends who sleep next to me and attend to my needs.

We watch Wasps winning the Premiership final together, and while I'm pleased for the lads, I can't help wishing I was there. Not long ago, Twickenham felt like a second home, now it feels like some distant, unreachable utopia. Then there's England's summer tour of New Zealand, which had been billed as me versus Dan Carter, the best fly-half in the world. We get beaten in both Tests, and Carter runs the show.

When my cast comes off, the doctor says I could be back playing in nine months. Kevin's not having that either, thinks I'll be back sooner. The first time I see him, I think he's just going to give my ankle the onceover. Instead he says, 'I've got to break down the scar tissue,' before really getting into it.

My God, it's the worst pain I've ever felt, like being driven over by a train. When Kevin's done torturing me, I tell him I've seen physios treat players with bad ankle injuries and they're not in any pain. Kevin replies, 'That's because they're not doing it properly.' After that, whenever Wasps' physios want to see me, I do the bare minimum, as Kevin's is the only advice I follow.

The first time I run on the treadmill, I break down crying. But those tears aren't of desolation, they're the last remaining doubts leaving my body.

You get crazy close to a physio when you suffer a bad injury. That's why the good ones are counsellors as well as magicians at fixing bodies. Kevin's a wise man who's experienced a lot and picked up plenty of knowledge from the people he's treated, who have ranged from old schoolmates to athletes and aristocrats. He's got a beautiful perspective on life, a great understanding of the world and a huge heart. And because Kevin treats my mind as well as my body, I'm back training with Wasps three months after the doc said I might be finished.

* * *

I'm 18 when I get my first proper girlfriend, a woman who's 30. When I tell her it's over, she tries to jump out of the car while it's moving. That scares me shitless. Since then, I've been reluctant to tell girls how I really feel in case they do something stupid. But there's more to my reticence than that.

My early interactions with women were innocent and enjoyable, but there came a time when I needed women like an alcoholic needs booze. Without women, giving me attention, making me feel wanted, I felt empty. Just sitting alone with my thoughts was difficult because I'd be wrestling with shame and self-loathing. So off I'd go again, searching for that hit, even though it was no longer providing me with the pleasurable feeling it once did.

Some of my mates are horrible, they'll drop women at a stroke, often with a brutal send-off – 'Fuck off, I don't wanna see you again.' That's not in my nature. I'm warm and kind, but that just makes women think I've fallen in love with them, when they're actually being manipulated, like counters in a game. I offer just enough to keep them on board, so they give me what I need, while keeping most of myself hidden.

Sometimes I talk to Kevin about women, while he's putting me through hell on the physio table. He'll say, 'Danny, you're a good-looking bloke, a professional athlete, just having fun. You've got nothing to feel bad about.' I get what he's saying, but even I can see that I'm an arsehole. I joke with my mates that I've got a squad of women 20 or 30 strong. I tell them I've got my star players and regular starters, and others who are usually on the bench but can do a decent job in an emergency. That sort of stuff is said in jest, and it makes my mates laugh. But even as I'm saying it, I know it's wrong.

Blokes will say, 'What a load of bollocks, how can sleeping with that many women make you unhappy?' But lots of things that start out as innocent fun can end up making you unhappy. I'm looking for love, but even I don't know where parts of myself are hidden, so what hope do I have of finding it? The truth is, I'm drifting further and further from love the more I search.

I meet Kelly while I'm recovering from my injury, at a computer game convention in London. As I'm arriving, she's leaving with her manager, who happens to be a big rugby fan.

I kind of recognise her, think I must have seen her on TV. More importantly, she's stunning. As for me, I'm 20 years old, an England rugby player, and I've got so much confidence you can almost see it coming out of my pores. So I chuck Kelly a few lines and give her my number.

For the next couple of months, we're inseparable. Kelly is the first girl I've fallen in love with, so now when I'm with my mates I don't make jokes about my squad of women, because it's been disbanded. We manage to keep a lid on our relationship, until we're spotted leaving a restaurant in the West End. By the autumn, we've moved in together.

Everything's coming at me thick and fast around this time. There's been the fiasco before the Scotland game, replacing Jonny as England's golden boy, swearing on TV, the injury, and now I'm dating a celebrity. As far as the tabloids are concerned, this is the icing on the cake. If I'm dating a celebrity, that must make me one, which means I'm fair game in their eyes.

I'm still only 20, so I'm not thinking, *Do I really want to be entering that celebrity world?* I like this woman and she likes me, that's the end of it. I'm quite innocent really, don't know how that world works. But I soon find out. Every time I leave our house in Notting Hill, there's paparazzi outside. They take photos of me removing parking tickets from my windscreen (admin has never been my thing). They take photos of me strolling to the shops. The lengths they'll go to, just to get a snap of me doing the most mundane things, is insane.

Suddenly, I'm all over the papers. Even the rugby writers are calling me a playboy, a man about town, and suggesting it's all gone to my head. As usual, it's Shaun Edwards who cuts through all the nonsense. 'If I could have pulled a bird like that when I was 20,' he tells journalists, 'I would have.'

Maybe I don't always do myself any favours. Because here I am, having my photograph taken with three half-naked women draped over me. But I'm only doing it because they asked me. I didn't think, *What's the correct thing to do here? What's the right way to behave? Will this come across wrong, portray me in a bad light, leave me open to criticism?* I'm not that calculating, I'm just going with the flow, doing what feels natural, what looks fun.

Plus, I thought I could show rugby in a different, more modern light. How many rugby players do you see on the cover of newspaper magazines? And it's not the *News of the World*, it's the *Observer*, an upmarket, sensible broadsheet, and there's also a good, in-depth interview.

As it happens, it's not fun, it's awkward. I don't stroll into the studio and start barking demands. I'm super tense and the models aren't talking to me, let alone trying to tear my clothes off. But people are always saying rugby doesn't market itself properly and at least I'm doing my bit.

What people don't know is that I'm turning down endorsement opportunities left, right and centre. The *Sun* offers me 80 grand to write a column, but I don't fancy it. Brylcreem offer me 100 grand, but I don't fancy that either. Nike offer me almost £1 million plus bonuses, but when Adidas counter with an offer of 700 grand over four years, I stay with them out of loyalty. Adidas have been giving me boots since I was 15, and I prefer theirs anyway, so it's a no-brainer.

If I was a guy with an out-of-control ego, I'd be saying yes to all these things. Maybe once I've done what I need to do, I'll be ready to make hay. For now, I'm a serious athlete, and I don't think I've done enough in the game to warrant those kinds of endorsements. Me and my agent part company in the end, because I'm the only client he's ever had who doesn't seem bothered about money, and I'm not happy with the direction he's trying to take me in.

Four months and three weeks after surgery, I'm starting for Wasps against Bath, the team we were playing when I knackered my ankle. That kind of recovery doesn't happen if you spend all your time out on the town, being a celebrity, it only happens if you're killing yourself every day to get better.

I last 53 minutes before being cheered from the pitch, having landed four of five kicks and had a hand in one of our tries. We lose, but I'm just relieved to come through without any of the metal in my ankle coming loose.

But just a week later, I'm all over the papers for the wrong reasons. The way they tell it, Josh Lewsey had a go at me for missing tackles in training, I gave him some lip back, and he knocked me out. The *Mirror*'s got the headline, 'FLASH DAN WALLOP'. Because *he* punched *me*, and he's a World Cup legend and they've decided I'm an arrogant celebrity, it's assumed I was being disruptive and he rightfully took me down a peg. But that's not true.

This is how it actually went down. Shaun had asked me to lead the session and Josh was having a nightmare, as he often does in training. I can't remember exactly what I said – other than it being a few stern words of advice, like Kingy used to dole out from time to time – but the next thing I knew, I was waking up in the physio room with smelling salts under my nose.

I've no idea who leaks their version of the story to the papers, but it's pretty poor form. Now everyone thinks it was all my fault and that I'm not a team man, whereas the truth is I gave Josh a bit of stick and he hit me. The irony is, I'm meant to be the one who needs to grow up, and Josh, a 35-year-old team veteran, is the one who's thrown a toddler's tantrum.

The media run with this story for days. I've got reporters firing questions at me when I leave the house, paparazzi wanting pictures of my cut lip, and I'm thinking, *Is this for real? What other athlete has to put up with this rubbish?* I even start thinking that maybe I've remembered it all wrong, that I did have that punch coming, that I do deserve all this negative attention.

Shaun barely mentions it, because he sees a bit of conflict as a positive thing. And it's not like we all have a summit to discuss our feelings. But the way I see it, we need to get past it quickly, because we've got a game on Saturday, against Castres in the Heineken Cup.

I ask Josh if he's ever seen *Remember the Titans*, which is a film about high school American football, containing a scene in which the two captains shadow box, swing at each other and then hug. 'If either of us scores this weekend,' I say, 'that's our celebration.' Sure enough, when Josh goes over for a try, we do the routine. And it's hugs again on the final whistle. I think that's a pretty savvy bit of diplomacy for someone who's not meant to be a team man.

9

EVERYTHING JONNY ISN'T

Jonny's dislocated his knee, so I suppose Martin Johnson doesn't have much choice but to rush me back into action. But I'm still surprised to be included.

Turning up to the England training camp for the autumn internationals, it feels like I'm almost back to square one. Towards the end of the previous season, I'd been ripping up teams for fun in a Wasps shirt. After the Ireland game, people thought I was destined to lead England into a dashing new era. Then came my injury, Brian's sacking and a new coach with an unknown philosophy.

A week into Johnno's first training camp and I still can't tell what his philosophy is. It's as if the RFU thought him just being Johnno would be enough, that players would naturally absorb his Johnno-ness by osmosis.

What does Johnno really know about how to play rugby? He spent his whole career with his head down in the middle of melees, hitting rucks, pushing in scrums, jumping in line-outs. If you think of rugby as a painting, Johnno knows his corner of the canvas intimately, but he can't possibly understand the full picture. If I had to guess, his philosophy is something along the lines of making his pack as tough as possible, because there's a lot of brutal high-contact training with forwards coach John Wells.

One thing I do know for certain, Johnno doesn't want me to run things like Brian did. There are no conversations, I'm just being spoken at. But I'm just happy to be back playing with England, so I'll sit back and see if I can figure things out.

I come through our first game against the Pacific Islanders unscathed, and score a try, but we don't exactly set the world alight. And before the game against Australia, I get the sense that no-one really knows what they're doing.

It's two days before the game and we've been training for two and a half hours. Everyone's grumbling and I'm thinking, *We're playing Australia on Saturday and half my team's knackered. Why is everyone going along with this? Why is no-one saying anything?*

I say to the skipper Steve Borthwick, 'Mate, we've been out here for two and a half hours, it should be an hour max, two days before a game. Are you gonna say anything to Johnno?' Borthers replies, 'I think Johnno's just trying something.' I say, 'Trying something? Tell him to try something with the under-15s. We're all gonna be fucked on Saturday.' I don't think Borthers says anything to Johnno. Everyone just stomachs it, in the classic English way.

Running out at Twickenham, I still don't know what the system is. We've been provided with a script, which is to play two, three or four phases in advance. Unfortunately, there are 15 blokes on the other team determined to tear our script up and trample it to dust. That's the ultimate irony: we're organised to within an inch of our lives, but when things don't go to plan, as they don't a lot of the time, it all feels scarily disorganised.

Still, we're leading with half an hour to go, and I've managed a couple of line-breaks. But I mostly remember groans.

I've just come back from a terrible career-threatening injury and I've lost some confidence. Before the injury, I was hell for leather, would tear into anyone and anything with no fear. But since coming back, I've become conscious that I'm not as committed with ball in hand.

I used to be a massive running threat, defenders couldn't deal with my speed, but now I'm beating one man, reaching the next and backing off. And once you become conscious of something, you can't get it out of your head.

Plus, it's difficult to outshine your opposite number when no-one in your side knows what he's doing. I'm still learning the art of playing at 10, but I do know that it's about getting a grip on your team, and that if everyone knows his role and what the coach's vision is, everything falls into place.

We've got world champions South Africa next and the mood in the camp is bleak. I'm getting a kicking in the media and I could do with someone taking me aside and telling me they still believe in me, that I'm still young, that together we'll work things out.

It's not like Shaun is always putting his arm around me and whispering nice things into my ear, but I know he cares, because of the time he gives me. In contrast, Johnno and his coaching team are very old-school rugby people who don't really do personal relationships or emotional intelligence. There's no sense of empathy or understanding. And this is England, the pinnacle. Shocking really. Unsurprisingly, the Springboks slaughter us, scoring five tries to nil in a 42–6 win, which is England's biggest ever defeat at Twickenham.

If I have a coach who sees and values how I can play the game, like Brian and Shaun, and puts people around me that are on the same page, there's no opponent I'm afraid of. But on this occasion, I felt like the whole team was underprepared for the realities of international rugby.

I get panned in the media, for my tactical kicking, my defence, my general lack of a clue. According to some writers and pundits, it's suddenly clear I'm not a Test fly-half and it would be tantamount to cruelty to start me against the All Blacks the following week.

They're particularly fixated on a clearance kick that got charged down and led to a try. It's happened a few times recently, admittedly, but they're talking as if it's a permanent chink in my game. I think, *Don't worry, I know how to fix it, I just have to make a slight adjustment to the speed of the kick.*

I feel like I've been fed to the wolves. But when Johnno tells me I'm on the bench for the All Blacks game, I can't really complain.

Before the first Six Nations game against Italy in 2009, Johnno calls me to say I'm not in his future plans and that he's going in a different direction. The conversation gets a bit heated. I tell him it's not fair, ridiculous. But because I'm so shocked, and lack experience, I forget to ask him for concrete reasons.

After I hang up, I think of all the things I should have said. I've bust a gut to get back from a horrible injury, I still haven't rediscovered my best form. How can you write me off based on a couple of bad games? Why don't you tell me to go back to my club, that you'll be watching, that if I play well you'll bring me back in? Then I feel despair. He's made it quite clear I don't fit in, and never will, at least as long as he's in charge.

There's talk in the papers about bust-ups in Portugal. One was meant to be with attack coach Brian Smith, who apparently had me in a headlock. Another was meant to be with John Wells. John is a classic, hardnosed Leicester man, who just wants people to smash into each other and be tough guys. Do as you're told, put your body on the line, don't complain, and if you're not hobbling off the training ground, you haven't given your all. But there were no bust-ups. All I did is raise questions about the attritional nature of training.

Maybe if I'd done well in the autumn internationals, they would have let it slide. As it is, maybe they hope that if they label me disruptive, and leak some lies to the press, journalists will stop asking why I'm out of the picture.

There's also a story about me missing a meeting because I was in Milan for a fashion show. But there was no meeting, it was a weekend. And Shaun had given me permission to be there. 'Dinner with David Beckham?' he says, 'Yeah, get yourself over there.' I had a great time with David, so there are no regrets. But it feeds into the narrative that I've taken my eye off the ball, that I'm out of control, not taking my rugby seriously, more interested in being a celebrity than a professional athlete.

It doesn't matter how many times Shaun or Geech or my Wasps team-mates tell them how hard I work, because that's not a headline. It doesn't matter that whenever I'm seen leaving a restaurant, I've just been out for a bite to eat. It doesn't matter that other young rugby players are getting pissed most weeks. Journalists have established their narrative and they're sticking with it, because the lie is more exciting than the truth and likely to be read by more people.

Sometimes I think, *Everyone seems so confident they know who I am, maybe they're right? Maybe it's me who's deluded?* I've got no-one to advise me either way, because no rugby player has ever been through what I'm going through. Gavin Henson has the celebrity girlfriend, which makes him tabloid fodder, but he's celebrated in Wales and they love him there.

When England lose two in a row against Wales and Ireland, journalists and pundits start calling for me to be recalled. I'm playing some great stuff for Wasps, reckon I'm getting back to my best, and labelling me disruptive hasn't thrown people off the scent. Plus, none of those journalists and pundits know that Johnno's told me I'm surplus to requirements for the foreseeable future.

Wins over France and Scotland ease some of the pressure on Johnno, but I'm just trying to help Wasps qualify for Europe and catch the eye of the Lions coaching team, which happens to include Shaun and Geech. Wasps miss out on qualification by one place, but Geech keeps dropping hints to the press that they might fancy me as a bolter for the trip to South Africa.

When the Lions squad is named, I'm not in it. They're only taking two fly-halves, Ronan O'Gara and Wales's Stephen Jones. It stings a bit, because I thought I'd shown them enough at the back end of the season, and I can cover other positions. But Geech tells me to stay fit in case of injury and I trust him.

Johnno doesn't pick me for England's tour of Argentina either, even though Jonny and Toby Flood are injured. Instead, I'll be playing for the Saxons in Colorado. One rugby writer calls the decision vindictive, another calls it shameful, another calls it baffling.

When Johnno is asked to explain my omission, he gets bristly, says it's got nothing to do with my attitude but is simply down to the fact that I'm not playing well enough. Geech has got me on standby for the Lions, Johnno thinks I'm the sixth-best 10 in England.

I'm keeping myself fit, just in case, when I get a text from Shaun. 'Danny,' he says, 'are you fit?' I tell him I've been working with Margot, and that Kevin says my ankle's in pretty good shape. 'Good,' says Shaun. 'Halfpenny's struggling with an injury, he might not make it. Expect a call from Geech.'

Wales's Leigh Halfpenny was picked primarily as a wing, but I assume Shaun and Geech have called me because I can also cover full-back and fly-half, and they're having second thoughts about only taking two 10s.

When Geech calls, he tells me I'm on board, but also that he needs to speak to England first, because I've had a knock on my ankle and they have to sign me off fit. That won't be a problem, because I've been working hard with Margot and Kevin since the end of the season. And I'm already thinking, *Maybe if I impress in a couple of midweek games, like bolters often do, I'll sneak onto the bench for the Test team.* I call my mum and Dom Waldouck to tell them the good news. I don't think I've ever been more excited.

When England call me in for a fitness test, they don't mention anything about the Lions, so I assume they're making sure I'm okay for the Saxons. But the following day, Geech calls to tell me they can't take me to South Africa, because England say I'm unfit, and therefore the Lions' insurance won't cover me. Geech doesn't know what to say. Shaun calls later to apologise for messing me around. They're genuinely gutted for me, but there's nothing they can do.

How do I explain that feeling? Imagine the thing you've been dreaming about your whole life suddenly happens, and the following day it gets taken away.

When I get off the phone to Geech, I go mental. Going on a Lions tour was everything to me, and now England have pulled out all the stops to prevent it from happening. It's disgusting and I'm completely and utterly devastated.

I don't understand why Johnno didn't speak to me, or Kevin, or Margot. I can only imagine the RFU had a say in it, because I could have made them look ridiculous. Can you imagine, Johnno thinks I'm the sixth best fly-half in England and there I am with the Lions in South Africa, pulling up trees against provincial sides midweek and maybe forcing my way into the Test team. How could Johnno not pick me after that? Talk about being in an uncomfortable position.

Johnno tells the media it was the Lions' decision not to take me. Technically, he's right, but only because England told them I was unfit. That rugby writer was correct when he said things were getting vindictive.

But I'm not the sort of person who picks up the phone and pours my heart out to a journalist. It wouldn't be a good idea anyway. People already think I'm a misfit. If I go to the press and say anything against Martin Johnson – World Cup-winning captain, national hero – you can add 'traitor' to that list, and I'll probably never play for England again.

10

DARKNESS ENGULFS ME

A few days after the Lions' first game in South Africa, I play for the Saxons against Argentina B. Northampton's Stephen Myler replaces me in the second half, before Stuart Lancaster drops me for the game against America.

I'm also on the bench for the final against Ireland, which we lose handily. Afterwards, Lanny says to me, 'We should have put you on sooner.'

Me and a couple of the boys head to a club in Glendale, one of those places with women dancing on the bar, like in the film *Coyote Ugly*. We have a good night, but as we're leaving, there are camera flashes going off in my face. I think, *Jesus Christ, I've come all the way to Colorado and they're still on my case.*

The photographer legs it, so me and a mate chase him down, grab his camera and remove the memory card. The police turn up and threaten to pepper spray us. I say to them, 'So it's okay for him to stick a camera in my face and take photos without my permission?' And they tell me it's not against the law.

A couple of days later, the photographer writes a story in the *News of the World*, justifying his harassment. He claims that because I don't mind being snapped coming out of The Ivy with my girlfriend, I have to expect to attract interest in other places. When did I say I don't mind? Of course I mind, because every time it happens, it gets added to the RFU file marked: 'REASONS WHY DANNY CIPRIANI SHOULD NOT PLAY FOR ENGLAND.'

It's quite a thick file, but it mainly contains stories about me going out for nice dinners. But in a sport obsessed with keeping up appearances, it's a very damaging one.

There's something missing at Wasps when we return for the 2009–10 season. When Lawrence retired in 2008, it felt like the heart had been ripped out of the club. And now Lewsey, Haskell, Tom Palmer, Tom Voyce and Eoin Reddan, all internationals and proven winners, have followed him out the door. That's the problem with the salary cap, it makes it impossible to build a dynasty, because the longer a trophy-winning player stays at a club, the more he expects to earn.

Geech has gone, too, and he was a genuine bloke who demanded respect. Meanwhile, Shaun is spending a lot of time away with Wales. I wouldn't say he's taken his eye off the ball, but his energy is often elsewhere.

Sadly, the other coaches don't possess his strength of personality. Tony Hanks, Geech's replacement as director of rugby, used to be our analyst and knows the club well. I like Tony, and he has some great ideas, but he isn't able to galvanise a group and conjure energy like Shaun can.

We start the season well, until the injuries kick in. Our skipper Tom Rees knackers his shoulder, Phil Vickery knackers his neck, hooker Rob Webber knackers his knee, and Simon Shaw and Joe Worsley are out as well. When I fracture my fibula in a win over Northampton, the papers reckon it's scuppered my chances of an international recall. What they don't know is that Johnno wouldn't have picked me even if I was the last fly-half in England.

I don't watch the autumn internationals, but apparently England were dismal. Jonny's playing some of the best rugby of his career with Toulon, so Johnno's recalled him, but it's the same old story in the media – England need a creative spark, England need a bit of magic. Maybe England need Cipriani.

But in early 2010, Wasps aren't even sure if they need me. Dave Walder played well at fly-half while I was out injured, and when I make my return against Harlequins at Twickenham, I miss five out of seven kicks. So now I've been taken out of the firing line, switched to full-back while Dave stays at 10. He's not a better player than me, but it makes sense. They need some stability, someone who's going to kick the ball a lot and not do anything complicated.

I'm still not the same player I was before my ankle injury. I've lost the explosiveness and excitement factor that made people sit up and take notice. I'm not taking the line on, which means I'm less likely to create space for others. I need to work out a new way to play the game and run a team.

That's not going to happen the way my mind is. I'm trying to prove a point every time I step onto a field, which is physically and mentally draining. All the negative things they're writing and saying about me are starting to take a toll. I've got more doubt now than I've ever had, and the magic comes when you're having fun, doing things without thinking, rather than trying to force it.

The bullshit is coming thick and fast. Former England captain Will Carling writes a blog claiming that when we met, I made it clear I wasn't bothered about playing for England.

Not bothered about playing for England? He couldn't be more wrong, because being seen as the best has been an obsession of mine since I was a kid. What I actually told him was that since achieving my dream, the energy had changed, and that even thinking about England was proving painful.

One ex-England player claims I'm an outcast at Wasps, slinking in and out of the place, moping about in training. Another claims I've lost the respect of my teammates. Maybe someone in the team is leaking this stuff, but whoever it is and whatever his motives, it's just not true.

I'm not the player I was, I've drifted miles from England selection, and people are writing shit about me in the papers every day, so it's hardly surprising I'm a bit withdrawn and struggling to focus on my game. But do you really think Shaun would keep picking me if I'd downed tools? Would Wasps be trying to get me to sign a contract extension?

Problem is, we've still got a stack of experienced England players and the new owners are unwilling or unable to pay them what they deserve. They even say to us, 'Take it or leave it. Don't bother involving your agents because we're not negotiating.' They make me feel like I'm being treacherous for even thinking about leaving, based on the fact that I came through their academy.

Even people who are meant to be my friends are spouting nonsense about me. In his column, Lawrence Dallaglio says I'm always going to be harder work than Jonny Wilkinson because I come with baggage and everything came to me too easily. If Lawrence had picked up the phone and called me, I'd have told him that just because someone is different, it doesn't mean they're hard work, not if you take the time to get to know them. I'd have said, I thought rugby was meant to be inclusive, 'a game for everybody', so why am I being portrayed as a misfit, someone who needs to be hammered into a certain shape? The same shape as Jonny Wilkinson.

As for his claim that my natural talent has made me complacent, Lawrence doesn't know what I had to go through as a kid, how I virtually brought myself up, how much harder than other kids I worked. If he'd asked, I'd have told him about my sprint sessions with Margot – catching the 4.30 train to Guildford after school, arriving at 5.30, training until 7, getting home at 8.30, all paid for out of my own pocket. But he didn't ask. Nobody did.

* * *

Previously, the rugby field felt like my safe space. Now, it's just another place where I'm being judged and critiqued. So I'm not exactly the life and soul in training, and I'm grinding through games with all the joy of a factory worker.

It's when I'm on my own that the darkness engulfs me. I feel like a wounded animal in his den, hoping no-one will smell blood and finish me off. Never wanting to leave, but also worried that the roof will fall in and bury me.

I've bought a place in Wimbledon, but the bastard paparazzi have tracked me down. Just after moving in, I was driving here from Kelly's place in Notting Hill when I clocked three cars behind us. I drove all the way around the M25 to try and lose them, but when I pulled over on the hard shoulder, they pulled up behind me, before following me the whole way home.

Shaun looks out for me, and we discuss a lot of things, but talking about mental illness is another thing entirely. Shaun's got a lot on his plate, what with Wasps and Wales, and I have a deep sense of shame for feeling how I do.

Mum and Dad have never sat me down and given me advice. Worse, Mum pores over social media, fan forums and the comments sections of newspaper articles, and she believes all the negative stuff she reads.

Most mums are fiercely defensive of their children, even if the bad stuff that's being written about them is true. But it feels like my mum is the opposite. She rants and raves down the phone – 'WHAT THE HELL HAVE YOU DONE NOW?' – and when I tell her it's all made up, she refuses to believe me. It's hard to think that Mum would believe the media over her own son.

Kelly's got her own life and doesn't do deep and meaningfuls. Sometimes, I think the only thing we have in common is that we both feel under siege. Every time she breaks up with me, which is often, it feels like the life's been sucked from me. When we get back together, it's the same old problems. As long as we're spotted leaving some posh restaurant or bar together, that seems to be enough for her. But getting spotted leaving posh restaurants is who she is, whereas it's not what I ever wanted to be.

Every time I leave the house, I think people are looking at me and judging. I can't go out and have a quiet drink with my mates because bar owners call the paparazzi. Mercifully, I've got a good friend called Malcolm who owns a nightclub in Soho. He sneaks me in through the back entrance, gives me a private booth and makes sure the coast is clear when I leave.

In Malcolm's club, I meet the guy who can get me a gun. I'd known him a while and thought he was straight up and wouldn't betray me. I'm driving when I get the call from my agent. 'Listen,' he says, 'the *Sun* are running a front-page story, saying you're trying to buy a gun. What the fuck is going on?'

My whole body is tingling. That'll be panic and fear. The guy must have ratted me out because I kept messing him around. Must have thought, *This geezer's all over the place, he's never gonna pay me for this gun, so I'll sell all his messages to the* Sun *and make a few quid.*

I don't want people to know the truth, that I'm weak and messed up and I want to end it all. So I speak to Damian Hopley from the Rugby Players' Association. He puts me in touch with his brother Phil, who's a psychiatrist, and Phil tells the *Sun* it would be highly unethical to run a story about a man who's undergoing treatment for his mental health. I'm not confident the *Sun* will take any notice, but, to my enormous relief, the editor spikes the story.

If that guy hadn't called the *Sun*, who knows how things would have panned out. I've always been impulsive, and suicide seemed like the only way out, so there's a chance I would have gone through with it. Maybe he did me a favour by grassing me up. As much as it scared the life out of me, it sent me down the right path. I'll be forever grateful to Phil for giving me the chance to speak out loud for the first time in my life, to put words and pictures to how I was feeling. It was like he'd pulled me out of that den just before the roof fell in.

MARGOT WELLS

When Danny's mum phoned and asked if I'd coach him, my reaction was, 'Urgh, not interested.' I'd had enough of coaching rugby players and being blamed for everything that went wrong with them. But I told Danny to ask his coaches at Wasps and see what they said. His coaches told him not to work with me, but he ignored them and I started coaching him anyway.

The first time I met Danny, I picked him up from Guildford railway station in his school uniform. I wasn't even out of the carpark when he said, 'We're going to get on, because we're both the same.' I thought, *That's quite astute for a 17-year-old.*

No-one who knew Danny would ever question his commitment to anything, especially not rugby. He'd go straight from school to train with Wasps, then come straight to me. I'd pick him up and drop him off again after training, and we did that day after day until he left school.

There was always something different about Danny. He had phenomenal, God-given talent, but still had the desire to make himself better, which says a lot about a person. He was very mature in how he saw the game and how he saw training. And he was always asking questions: 'Why are we doing this?' 'What will it do?' 'How will it help?' Most kids aren't like that.

There are athletes who are gifted a perfect functioning body at birth – think Roger Federer and how he moved – and Danny had that. But before I started working with him, that had been taken away in the weights room.

I always say, 'If you can't make somebody faster, for God's sake don't make them slower.' Making somebody slower should be a criminal offence. So we got back to making Danny's body function how it was meant to function.

All my players do their own thing, because not everybody's got the same body. But Danny once said to me, 'Why does everybody else in the squad do the same exercises every day?' I replied, 'Because they weren't gifted the bodies that you were gifted.' Then he rang me up and said, 'Margot, I'm doing the same exercises as everybody else on team runs and match days.' I replied, 'That's all well and good, but that means you're training with one body and playing with a different one.' Danny said, 'But I like some of them.' And I replied, 'Well, do the ones you like, and don't do the ones you don't like.'

A whole team doing the same exercise programme is madness. And if a player needs to do certain things because it makes him feel good, and contribute to the game in a positive way, what's the problem?

To answer my own question, the problem is the coaches' egos, and their ignorance, in both senses of the word. They know their way, and no other way. And if anybody challenges their way, they don't want to listen.

Too many coaches think they're due respect simply because they're coaches. But you have to earn Danny's respect, he won't just give it to you. That's why he never made the 2019 World Cup. They just made up that he wasn't fit, the real reason was that they couldn't cope with Danny, someone who knew more about rugby than them, being in the squad. If they'd had any brains in their heads, they would have let Danny get on with what he had to do and taken all the glory when it reaped rewards.

Sometimes it seems like English rugby wants everybody to be average, like it doesn't want anybody to stand out. It's like the players have all come out of the same factory, and not a great one. Look at the way England play the game. Who would you be frightened of in the current England team? But when Danny was available, someone who thought outside of the box, who had the amazing ability to see things nobody else did, they hammered him.

I wasn't just Danny's sprint coach, we also worked on his mind, because you can't separate the two. So I was aware of everything that was going on, on and off the field, and how all that public scrutiny affected him.

I knew how the British press worked, because of what they wrote about me and my husband [former Olympic 100m champion Allan Wells] that wasn't true. I remember saying to Danny, 'The press are jealous of your ability and who you sleep with. They have a story they want to write, and if you confirm that, fair enough. But if you don't, they're going to write it anyway.'

All Danny wanted to do was play rugby, and he worked so hard to be the best he could for the team, whatever that team was. So it saddens me that he wasn't allowed to enjoy the fruits of his labour, that he was labelled a 'bad boy' when he was actually a great kid. People say he didn't always help himself, and maybe he didn't. But no-one should have to put up with that kind of abuse.

Danny still comes and trains with me, when he's not travelling the world taking pictures of himself. You should see him interacting with kids at the track, he introduces himself to all of them and they're completely in awe of him. Kids need role models, and he could still be a role model for rugby if they'd let him, because he's got so much to contribute.

While I always say that part of my job is to make dreams come true, and I'm happy to admit I made a huge difference to certain players' careers, I just feel privileged that Danny allowed me to be part of his.

It's great that he seems to have come to terms with things that happened. Danny's a good friend, and he deserves some peace in his life.

11

DESPERATELY WANTING TO FEEL

An old agent of mine tells me they're starting up a new Super Rugby franchise in Melbourne and they want me to come and play for them. I've had a few offers from French clubs, and that's where everyone expects me to go, but now I'm thinking, *I've always loved southern hemisphere rugby, and their club competition is the best. You know what? Melbourne makes a lot of sense.*

Rod Macqueen's going to be head coach of Melbourne Rebels, which worries me slightly. Rod was in charge of Australia when they won the 1999 World Cup but hasn't coached anyone for almost a decade. That's a long time in rugby. But when I'm told some of the other players Melbourne are after – former Wallabies Stirling Mortlock and Mark Gerrard, former All Blacks prop Greg Sommerville, Tongan wing Cooper Vuna, who's switching from Australian rugby league and has a highlights reel to die for – I'm excited.

And I haven't been excited about anything for quite a while.

I've also discovered that no-one gives a shit about rugby union in Melbourne, which is probably why no-one's thought of putting a club there before now. That makes it an even more attractive proposition, because I'll be able to let my hair down and have fun without being badgered and judged, and hopefully start feeling like my old self again.

Johnno won't be able to pick me for England, due to the RFU's rules. But even if I'd stayed at Wasps and performed miracles, he'd have been unmoved. So I'm not going to keep banging my head against a brick wall, and Melbourne sounds like a healthier escape than a bullet to the head. Plus, even if I stay there for two years, I'll still only be 24 when I return, a better player for the experience and with three seasons to get back into contention for the 2015 World Cup. And hopefully Johnno will be gone by then.

Shaun and Tony don't want me to leave, but they understand. They know how down I've been and want me to be happy. Not that I get much of a send-off. I'm on the bench for my last home game, a loss to Cardiff in the Amlin Cup semi-finals, and I break my thumb in my last Premiership game against Newcastle. Not to worry, I've got five months off before I have to be in Melbourne.

Wasps team-mates George Skivington and Rob Hoadley have been spending their summers in Los Angeles for the last few years. When they turn up at pre-season, they show me photos of the women they've been shagging and I can't get my head around it. George is a tall good-looking fella, and Rob's handsome enough, but these girls are off-the-scale stunning, like *Sports Illustrated* swimsuit models.

I say to them, 'Lads, there's no way on God's earth you're shagging these women.' They assure me it's happening, and I reply, 'But you two are schmucks. Who are you telling them you are? Prince William and Prince Harry?'

In the summer of 2010, I decide to go with them, along with a few other Wasps lads. But first me and Kelly spend a bit of time in Vegas. That doesn't go well. One night, we're in a strip club, pretty drunk, but still having a good time. But when I go off for a private dance, I start coming out with all this cheesy chat – 'Listen, I'm breaking up with her in LA, but I'll be back in Vegas next week' – the sort of pathetic bullshit the stripper's heard a thousand times before.

The stripper goes to the toilet, and a few minutes later, I clock Kelly marching towards me looking extremely annoyed. Before I have time to say anything, she slaps me across the face. Security come swarming, there's a big kerfuffle, and Kelly is eventually chucked out, arms and legs flailing.

Turns out Kelly overheard the stripper talking about me in the toilet – 'This English guy called Danny has just given me his number' – and decided I needed to be punished. I had a lot going on, and it was quite an immature relationship. But it was still despicable behaviour on my part, and I can't really blame her. I head to the toilet and take a piece of broken glass to my wrist. I'm not intending to end it all, I just desperately want to feel something.

LA is unbelievable – the boys aren't lying about the women – and after a week or so, Kelly has to return to

England for some photoshoot or other. When she asks if I'm coming with her, I say, 'Absolutely not, this is great.'

She storms off to the airport. And a couple of days later, she calls to say she's breaking up with me. It's happened hundreds of times before, but on this occasion, I'm not particularly bothered.

The following night, I meet a girl who's a dead ringer for Megan Fox, except better looking. Within minutes, I'm professing my undying love. She works as a bottle girl in a nightclub and makes a fortune in tips. There are NFL and NBA players throwing wads of cash at her, it's all over the floor like confetti. But when she clocks off for the night, it's me who goes back to her place.

I've been hammered for two days straight when I rock up to a house party we've been invited to. When I walk in, I feel a group of girls turn and look at me (I've always had excellent peripheral vision). One of my mates says, 'Do you know who that was who just checked you out?' I don't have a clue. 'That was Lindsay Lohan,' he says, as in the Hollywood actress.

I have a bit of a wander, head upstairs, and bump into Lindsay on the landing. It's her birthday the next day, so she invites me to hers. While I'm there, I call the lads and tell them to meet me at such and such apartment. They ring the bell, I go down and get them, and when they walk into the apartment, Lindsay's standing there in just a towel. She says hello and goes off to get changed, and they're all rooted to the spot with their jaws on the ground.

Later, we head to the club where the Megan Fox look-alike works. We haven't been there long when the Megan

Fox lookalike marches towards us and punches Lindsay in the face. I can't say for sure, but I think I'm to blame.

Only when I'm alone again in London does reality kick in. I'd planned on moving to Melbourne with my first love, and that's now up in smoke. I'm not in control of any part of my life, everything's slipping away from me.

When I close my eyes, I see myself as a kid, tearing down the stairs, bawling my eyes out, trying to catch up with my dad. And I feel that pain again, like part of my heart has been torn out.

Kevin seems to treat every famous person in the country, and it's through him that I meet Jamie Redknapp. I tell Jamie I'm at a loose end until I head to Melbourne, that I need to keep myself fit away from a rugby environment, and he suggests I train with Tottenham, who are managed by his dad Harry.

For six weeks, I travel an hour each way to Chigwell and back. But I absolutely love it. Gareth Bale is even better close up, and they've got a Moroccan kid called Adel Taarabt who can do ridiculous things with a ball. There's also a big English striker called Harry Kane who looks half-decent.

My positioning is all over the place, but my touch is as good as anyone's. So Harry asks if I fancy going to Spain with the Under-23s. It's not a PR stunt, because no-one really knows about it, and I end up playing at left-back against Valencia and Malaga.

Now I've got a bit of a bug, am intrigued to see how far I can go, so I train with QPR for a fortnight. I love the skills and attacking drills, not so much learning to defend. Movement in rugby is mainly side to side, while a footballer's movement is 360°, so when I play against West Ham, I'm a bit out of my depth. Frank Nouble's playing up front for West Ham, and he's not the most agile, but all he has to do is push the ball past me and I'm left for dead.

I then train with MK Dons, who are down in League One and a bit more my level. When Karl Robinson, their manager, asks what position I play, I tell him I play up top. On day one, the ball's played into me and I've got my back to goal and a centre-back right up my arse. I take a touch, bump the centre-back off with my shoulder, drag the ball back, flick it through his legs, go round him and play the ball in for someone to score. Karl likes what he sees.

At the end of the week, I have a discussion with Karl about signing a contract. And on the train home, I'm seriously thinking about sacking off Melbourne and joining MK Dons instead.

But the more I think about it, the less sense it makes. I love playing football, especially the changing room vibe. It's not so much that I prefer the people, more that I feel less constricted. Then again, there's no pressure on me to perform. I also think that if football doesn't work out, rugby won't accept me back. I'm already seen as an outcast, and they'll view this as the ultimate insult. And the bottom line is, I still want to play for England, perform on the biggest stage. Wise up, Danny, get yourself over to Melbourne and do what you've got to do.

I'm actually quite excited to get there. I'll be single, on the other side of the world, sounds like it could be a lot of fun. But there are negative vibes around me even before I fly out. According to the papers, Rod Macqueen's got the hump because I've been playing football. Then there's a delay with my visa, which means I miss a Rebels pre-season press conference. I have to hold my hands up, my fault completely. I've always been terrible at admin. It feels like conforming, like I'm being made to jump through hoops.

It's the morning of my flight and I haven't even packed. Part of me is thinking, *Australia? It's not exactly around the corner*. I drag a big bag from the wardrobe, stuff it with clothes and head to the airport.

12

FUCKED UP AGAIN

It's not exactly the warmest of welcomes. There's no, 'Welcome to Australia! You're going to love Melbourne! You're going to have a great time playing for the Rebels!' It's more like enlisting in the army. Lots of principles rammed down throats, this is what we stand for, you need to stand for the same.

The boys seem cool though. There's a bit of banter, but they don't seem to have formed an opinion about me based on what's been said in the media.

I've got a top-floor apartment in South Yarra, Melbourne's upmarket quarter. But I'm already at loggerheads with Rod. Because he hasn't coached for years, he's got something to prove, thinks he's going to reinvent the game. All hail Messiah Macqueen!

It doesn't feel very forward-thinking, the amount of running we're doing in pre-season. It's giving me tendonitis in my knees. In one session, Rod has us doing a 1 km time trial. We train with the ball for 15 minutes, then do a bleep test. We train with the ball for another 15 minutes, then do another 1 km time trial. Everyone's fucked.

We've got this rugby league conditioner who's very stats-orientated. 'Mate,' he'll say, 'fuckin' run this far, this fast, and I fuckin' promise you, mate, we'll be the fittest fuckin' team in the comp.' Which is, of course, nonsense.

It's important to be fit, but you've got to tailor fitness training to your sport. You've also got to keep in mind that if players enjoy what they're doing, train with smiles on their faces, they'll get through loads of work anyway, while improving their ability to make crucial decisions while fatigued.

Think back to when you were a kid, running around all day from dawn 'til dusk. You never went to bed thinking, *Blimey, I feel awful.* You felt nicely tired. And the following day, you did the same all over again. You could do that for weeks on end, because all that exercise was connected to having fun.

But in rugby, instead of fun being central to training, it's all 'DRILLS, DRILLS, DRILLS, GET FITTER, GET STRONGER, GET TOUGHER, GET MEANER.' Why? Because stuff like that is easy for coaches to quantify, while measuring a player's intuition, reading of the game and appreciation of space takes intelligence and time.

Rod wants to use more rugby league-style attacks, which intrigues me, because those boys can teach us a few things about running lines. But we end up doing some of the dumbest shit I've ever been involved in.

In one of our first meetings, he comes up with a move that has me thinking he's lost his mind. Off a line-out, he wants the inside-centre to carry and hit up, before everyone else, including the wingers and full-back, joins in a pick and go. He's even given this move a name, 'apple'. I can tell everyone's non-plussed, but nobody says anything.

I say to Stirling Mortlock, 'Mate, this move is madness,' and Stirling replies, 'You know Rod's a bit nuts but we'll give it a go.' I'm thinking, *You played 70-odd times for the Wallabies, you're our captain, and you're just gonna do what you're told, even though you know it's bullshit?*

When we get on the training field and try it for the first time, everyone does it but me. I say to Rod, 'I'm not doing that. First, what if the ball gets turned over? We're all in the middle of the field, so all they have to do is shift it wide and we're stuffed. Second, we're practising against bags, and whenever you pick and go against a bag you make three to five metres per pick. But when you pick and go against real defenders in a game, they actually resist.'

Afterwards, the younger lads are all taking the piss. 'What the fuck was that move? Apple! Crock of shit.' But no-one else says anything to the coaches.

Maybe I should be like the others, keep my head down and do what I'm told. But following orders without debate makes no sense to me. Not only does it make you a robot, it also leads to bad outcomes, especially if the orders are coming from a man who doesn't seem to be seeing clearly.

If I'd had a normal father-son relationship, maybe I wouldn't question things as much. As it is, I never really had to follow orders as a kid, I was making my own decisions from a young age. And if you do try to tell me what to do, and it makes no sense to me, I'll do my own thing instead.

I've also been spoilt in terms of coaches, because I could always discuss things with Brian and Shaun. But most rugby coaches aren't like them. Most rugby coaches seem to think that if they allow players to air opinions, they'll end up looking stupid and weak. That's why so many coaches are suspicious of people like me and seek to paint me as wilful, disruptive and disrespectful.

I'm on the bench for our first game against the Waratahs, which is the Rebels' Super Rugby debut and the first union fixture at AAMI Park. The UK papers are supportive as ever, the *Mirror* going with the headline 'DANNY DIRE' before I've even kicked a ball.

We try Rod's 'apple' move on our first or second play. Sure enough, we turn the ball over, they shift it wide and someone goes the length of the field and scores. Now I'm thinking, *Was I being defiant for the sake of it? Or was I being defiant because I thought it was best for the team?* Our starting fly-half Jimmy Hilgendorf gets injured after eight minutes, but there's not much I can do when our forwards are getting mangled, and the Waratahs hammer us 43–0. We get 25,000 fans watching us that night. I'm not sure many will be back.

That night, I'm in a club with some of the Waratahs boys – Kurtley Beale, Drew Mitchell and a few more of their young, dumb and very fun lads. I say to Drew, 'Let's play rock, paper, scissors. Loser has to nick that bottle of vodka from behind the bar.' One, two, three, draw ... One, two, three, fuck, I lose.

I'm pretty drunk and think I'm being sly. But no sooner have I swiped this bottle and stuffed it down my trousers than I feel a big paw on my shoulder. I spin around, see a giant bouncer staring down at me and can't stop giggling. The bouncer says, 'I've been watching you. What's that down your trousers?' I try to explain we're just messing around and that I'm going to put the bottle back, but the bouncer fails to see the funny side and boots us out.

I assume that will be the end of it, but the papers get hold of the CCTV footage, which is also played on the news, and the Rebels hit me with an official warning and a one-match fine.

I'm annoyed at myself for falling into the narrative that's been building, that I'm a loose cannon who doesn't give a shit. And while I understand why Rod and Stirling have to appear to take it seriously, put on their gravest faces and say things about it being a new club that needs to establish a squeaky-clean culture, perspective has gone out of the window. I'm a 22-year-old kid who's made a rash decision on a lads' night out, and the papers are talking about me as if I'm the second coming of Satan.

One of the papers back home claims my team-mates have nicknamed me 'Google', because I'm always googling my own name. I know what they're doing, they want readers to think my team-mates are calling me 'Google' because my ego is out of control. What actually happened was a few of us went to a nightclub and I forgot to bring ID, so one of the lads suggested I show the bouncers my Wikipedia page, which included my picture and date of birth.

There was a bit of banter on the back of that, with team-mates calling me Google in training, but it wasn't mean-spirited like that journalist made it out to be, and it only stuck for a couple of days. My actual nickname is 'Prince', because, for some bizarre reason, they think I sound like Prince Harry.

I've got a massive chip on my shoulder now, and I'm really quite angry, which isn't me at all. I feel horribly isolated, like I've been washed away at sea and have nothing to grab onto.

I get the feeling Rod never wanted me at the Rebels and that the decision to sign me was imposed on him from above. But with Jimmy injured, he doesn't have a choice but to start me for the next game against the Brumbies.

The Brumbies are packed with Aussie internationals, including Matt Giteau at fly-half, and expected to pummel us. But it's a tooth and nail affair from the off, a game in which anger comes in handy.

I score the Rebels' first ever points with a first-half penalty, Mortlock scores our first ever try with seven minutes left, but we're trailing by two points with 79 minutes on the clock. Then we get a penalty. It's not straightforward, on the 15-metre line and some way out, but I put everything into the kick and it sails between the posts. When the final whistle goes, my team-mates pile on top of me. They're smiling and screaming, and whatever they're feeling, I'm feeling it a thousand times over. Everyone had written us off, labelled us a joke, and now we've come out fighting and proved them wrong.

Unfortunately, a siege mentality will only carry you so far. There needs to be a deeper understanding, emotionally and technically, and I'm not sure we have the coaches to deliver that.

Rod's forwards coach, Mark Bakewell, is clearly hating the experience, wanders around the place like it's a funeral parlour. I don't have the knowledge to run a team, and Rod's never going to allow me to do that anyway. He wouldn't trust me to run a bath. To Rod I'm just a naughty boy. Whenever I ask a question, I can see him thinking, *God, here he goes again.*

We manage to string two wins together against Wellington's Hurricanes and Perth's Western Force, but it's mostly an uphill slog. We get smashed all over the southern hemisphere – in Brisbane, Sydney and Auckland, and usually at home as well.

On occasion, Rod will put me on the wing when we're defending, so the press have started calling me a liability. But here's the thing: the effectiveness of a team's defence is based on the energy a coach gives his players. If a coach clearly values me, I'll do anything for him. That's why Shaun never had any issues with my defence, and he was the best defence coach in the world.

I'm dropped to the bench for the game against the Waratahs in Sydney, before me and Richard Kingi get busted for breaking a post-match curfew. It's one thing after another.

It's not like I blame Shaun for my mistakes, but Wasps was my first experience of a professional environment, and it happened to be a successful one. It wasn't a free for all, far from it. But if someone did mess up, Shaun wouldn't react like it was the end of the world. His values were so deeply ingrained in the squad that bad things seemed to naturally correct themselves.

It doesn't help that Aussie athletes are looser than English ones, because the circumstances allow them to be. We play Friday nights, so have the whole weekend off. The sun is shining, the drink is flowing, every bar and pub has a stereo blasting and the women are barely clothed. I'm only 22, and never really did this stuff as a teenager, so of course I'm going to make the most of it.

My first night out in Melbourne, I'm offered cocaine. I was never aware of it in England, but over here it seems to be very popular, so I give it a go. I'm also introduced to sleeping pills and Red Bull, which gives you the sensation of being drunk and isn't going to get me into trouble. Or so I think. One morning, I wake up outside a takeaway, with a half-eaten kebab on my chest. I must have been there for a couple of hours. I only live about 50 yards away, so I brush myself down, wander home and fall into bed.

There's the training and the games, so I do feel like I've got a proper job, but I still need all that other stuff – the weekend drinking, the sleeping pills, the getting out of my mind, blacking out and not remembering how I got home – to fill the gaps. I feel like I'm scrabbling through life, constantly trying to put the pieces together.

* * *

I've seen pictures of Kelly and my old Wasps team-mate Thom Evans out and about at various West End night-spots which puts a giant dent in my ego.

Kelly and Thom are in every tabloid and all over the internet, so it's like my heart is being broken in glorious technicolour. It also feels like the ultimate betrayal, because Thom is meant to be a good friend. When I hear they're having a baby together, I'm devastated.

When Kelly starts messaging, implying she wants to get back with me, it messes with my head. When she loses the baby, we secretly meet up in Mauritius, while she's still meant to be with Thom. I know deep down it's wrong, but I'm convinced I want her back. I'm desperately grasping for remnants of my old life, because I think it will make me feel like the old me.

I've always felt alone, I'm used to it. But now I'm scared of being on my own for a second, because it means I might start thinking about my situation and fall into another depression. So I keep ploughing forward and ignoring reality. If I'm not playing rugby, I'm partying and getting intoxicated. And after I've finished partying and getting intoxicated, I'm having sex. It sounds like one hell of a life, but it's actually all proof that something's badly amiss.

I awake with a start and know straightaway that I've fucked up again. I look at my phone and the battery's dead. That means my alarm never went off and I've almost certainly overslept. A bunch of sleeping pills will do that to you.

I walk into my front room and find Peter Siddle, the Aussie fast bowler, crashed out on the couch. Unlike me, he's out of season and doesn't need to be anywhere. Peter lends me his car, I head for the training ground and soon hit traffic. I take the opportunity to close my eyes … when I open them again, probably only a few seconds later, I discover I've rolled into the car in front.

Having struck out three times, I'm axed from the squad for two games in South Africa. Some of my team-mates, experienced, solid family guys like Mark Gerrard and Luke Holmes who know what's what, look out for me, but no-one higher up says, 'Danny, what's going on? Are you okay, mate? Is there anything we can do to help?' Instead, it's, 'Mate, not again. Here's your punishment.'

I'm back for the last two games of the season, both losses. The Rebels' first season in Super Rugby hasn't been a roaring success, amounting to three wins, 13 losses and last place in the table. And it hasn't been the relaxing hiatus I envisaged. Anything that could go wrong has gone wrong. And I have to hold my hands up and say, *Mate, you can't keep blaming everyone else.*

13

SOME SEMBLANCE OF SERENITY

There's talk of me breaking my contract and heading back to England, but when the Rebels sack Rod and sign Wallaby superstars Kurtley Beale and James O'Connor, both serious talents, I want to stick around.

Besides, despite all the drama, I'm learning things. The South African sides are crazy physical, full of big, fast, direct runners. Aussie sides, maybe because of the rugby league influence, think outside of the box.

Kiwi teams play with freedom, are excited by the possibilities. Since they were kids, Kiwi players have been taught to do whatever feels right, not play to a set of orders. And because they have all the basic skills by the time they're adults, they have faith that if they move into the unknown and try something different, it's going to come off.

It's a far cry from English rugby culture, which is about certainty and control, knowing what players are going to do and fitting them into systems. If you crave certainty and control, need to know what's going to happen, you're missing out on what could happen. And what could happen might be wonderful.

I'm always picking up new tricks in Melbourne because I'm surrounded by people who love testing boundaries. After training, we set up grids and spend ages practising footwork.

Richard Kingi is a Kiwi and his footwork is unbelievable, he could sidestep you in a phone box. I notice that he jumps off one foot, and when he lands on the other, he'll read the defender's movement, step back inside and leave him for dead. Or he'll suddenly put in a goose step, which looks identical to a normal step until the last fraction of a second. Cooper Vuna, another Kiwi, has got machine gun feet – rat-a-tat-tat and he's gone. People think footwork is innate, but this is stuff Richard and Cooper were taught as kids, and now they're teaching it to me.

Luke Holmes, who's the third-choice hooker but much better than that, lives in a small apartment with his family, so I suggest we get a bigger house together and split the rent. Luke tells the bosses, and because he's a straight-as-a-die Christian man with a wife and two kids, they accept it as a solution.

I take the top floor, while Luke, Mel and the kids have the rest of the house to themselves. It's an unconventional arrangement, but it works a treat. Mel really looks after me, cooks and does my laundry. It's a lovely environment to be in, full of love and minus judgement. And because I don't want to betray their kindness, I rein in the wildness and discover some semblance of serenity.

But it's not like I suddenly turn into a monk. I go on a few dates with Miss Australia, which the papers obviously love. And in the summer of 2011, I find myself on a South Pacific island with a model who used to be engaged to the Australia cricket captain, which I think I've managed to keep a lid on.

We're staying in a house on stilts and it's ridiculously beautiful. I'm laid out on deck, drinking in the scene – crystal water, a sky that goes on forever, a setting sun that resembles a giant yolk dipping over the horizon, all that stuff you read in travel magazines – and then I hear this woman chatting on the phone. I think, *Who the hell is that? Why would she be talking to anyone?*

I listen more closely, catch the flow for a few seconds, and it sounds like she's chatting to a journalist. 'I think I love him, I'm so happy', that sort of stuff. Miffed, I walk inside and say, 'Are you doing an interview? Are you talking about me?' And she puts her hand over the phone and whispers, 'One second ...'

When she gets off the phone, she says, 'Are you cool with that?' I say, 'Not really.' We've got another three days on this island, so I try to bury my feelings, for the sake of having a good time. But after I get back to Melbourne, I never speak to her again.

Some weekends, a bunch of us gather at James O'Connor's rooftop apartment, which has a wraparound balcony, swimming pool, jacuzzi and barbeque.

I've known Kurtley since we were 17, when he was Australia's rugby prodigy and I was England's. Kurtley has a reputation for wildness, as has James. Chuck me into the mix and it's quite combustible. It's fun, but dangerous.

The upside is that I'm not in the news as much, because whenever I'm in a sticky spot, Kurtley and James are usually involved. It's one thing slagging off the Pom, another thing writing things that might harm the Australian team, especially with a series against the Lions on the horizon.

James works as hard as anyone, but he's a bit me, me, me on the field. James doesn't care who's in front of him, he's convinced he's going to beat them. He usually does, but there are times when he should be less selfish. James' confidence can curdle to recklessness when he's got a few drinks inside him, but he's a lovely bloke really, and we've got a lot in common. Like me and Kurtley, James was labelled a boy wonder. And like me and Kurtley, he had to figure himself out while under the gaze of a judgemental media and public.

I'm not sure Kurtley knows what he's doing half the time. He'll zig one way, zag another, and suddenly burst through a hole that didn't appear to be there. He's not smooth, like James, and always looks slightly out of control. But just when you think he's feinted himself into a corner, he'll find a way out.

I'd do anything for Kurtley, he's one of the good guys. When he's not drinking, he's quite reserved, but once alcohol touches his lips, oh boy, I've never seen such a dramatic transformation. Maybe we're drinking for similar reasons, because I know Kurtley had a tough upbringing. But with Kurtley, all those emotions he's bottling up react with the booze and come gushing out like a fountain, whereas with me, they stay locked away.

Me, James and Kurtley are three young men feeling the conformity of our sport – and our egos are out of control. We call ourselves 'The Big Three', as in Miami Heat's LeBron James, Dwyane Wade and Chris Bosh, and think we're going to take Super Rugby by storm. But that's not how it pans out.

Rod's replacement as head coach is Damien Hill, and he's more like a schoolteacher than a professional rugby coach. Then again, I imagine we're not particularly easy to handle.

Andrew Johns comes in and coaches us occasionally, and Shaun reckons he's one of the greatest ballplayers he's ever seen, in league or union. These top league guys seem to understand how to go to the line and open up space for others, in a way very few union players do.

Andrew is great on body position and disguising intent. Most fly-halves change their shape and angle depending on what they're going to do. For example, if they're going to throw a ball out the back, they'll turn sideways, which is a cue for the opposition to act. But Andrew teaches me to receive the ball in a position whereby the defence doesn't know if I'm going to run, kick, pass, play a short ball, a single miss, a long miss, or a ball out the back. That means defenders' feet are planted for a second or two longer, which makes all the difference at the elite level.

Andrew also talks to us younger players about the need to focus on our footy, and it feels real coming from him, because he's had plenty of controversy in his life. But he can't work miracles. Because we're playing in a system that isn't conducive to breaking down defences, me, James and Kurtley feel the need to do our own thing, instead of coming together and doing what's best for the team.

Besides, we keep getting injured. The first time all three of us start is in round seven, when we run Auckland's Blues ragged and win only our second game of the season. Two games later against the Waratahs, James lacerates his liver and is ruled out for six weeks.

A few of us break curfew after the Waratahs game – a night out in Sydney is too tempting to resist – and the club decide enough is enough. They don't want to make a big deal of it, as there's been enough negativity around the club already, so they put out a statement, explaining that it's amicable and I'm simply going home to prepare myself for the coming season in England, where I've signed a contract with Sale.

My time down under hasn't gone how I wanted it to, but I'm sad to be leaving Melbourne. I've made some great friends, people I'll stay in contact with for years to come. And I've learned a lot about rugby, even though there were a lot more losses than wins. That said, it's not as if I'm stepping into the unknown. It sounds like Sale really want me, as if I'll be seen and appreciated, which is all I ever wanted.

14

MY HEAD HURTS

I've got five months off before the Premiership season starts and I'm going to do whatever I want.

I've moved in with my old Rosslyn Park mate Rory Hamilton-Brown, who became a cricketer instead of a rugby player and is now captain of Surrey. Rory's got a big house in Wandsworth, bought by his dad, and it gets pretty heavy pretty fast. Lots of house parties, lots of girls – not a great lifestyle for professional athletes. But we're young, red-blooded men doing what young, red-blooded men do. At least that's what I tell myself.

I'm not the sort of bloke who swaggers into a pub or changing room and starts boasting about his latest conquest. But it's not exactly a secret I'm putting it about a bit. Thankfully, most of it doesn't make the papers.

When sex is one of the few things in your life that provides relief, you end up trying to find more and more unusual ways to get your hit. I'm sleeping with everyone from porn stars to actresses to girls I meet at the coffee shop. Threesomes have become the norm, but I just feel dejected when it's over. I don't allow myself to feel that for too long, though, and soon get back to distracting myself.

Whenever I move club, I start building up a new squad. I bring a few with me, the ones I want to spend time with, but most of the previous squad I cast adrift. It's not unusual for me to sleep with three different women in one day.

I have to be very disciplined with the timings, shuffling one girl out of the house just in time for the next one to turn up. If I suspect someone might tell stories, I won't reveal much of myself, will give them just enough to get what I want and nothing more. I have spells when I'm only having sex with women who are married or in a relationship, because I know they won't sell me out.

It may sound like every man's dream, but the art of life is finding the right balance. And in that respect, sex is no different to food or drink. While it's fine to like food and drink, if you like them too much, they can make you deeply unhappy and destroy your life.

Sex for me has become a form of self-harm. I can't do without that feeling sex gives me, but I'll often wake up in the morning and think, *Fucking hell, I certainly don't feel happier*. Occasionally, I think I'm in love. But a few weeks later, I won't want to be anywhere near them, which tells me this thing I'm chasing isn't love at all.

Life in Wandsworth is all a bit dark and dingy, and it strikes me that at least some people we're hanging around with are seeking respite from their own mental anguish – I know I am.

I often find myself talking through the night with Tom Maynard, Rory's Surrey team-mate who also lives with us. Tom's having a great year with the bat and being tipped to play for England. He's a top guy – funny, intelligent, mischievous, and a big-hearted lover of life.

One day in June, we hit the town. It soon gets messy and it's all a bit of a blur, but I'm sure it's been fun. We all head to bed at about 6 a.m., Tom on the top floor, me on the floor below, Rory across the landing. When I wake up the following morning, it's to the news that Tom has been hit by a train and killed.

Tom's death makes no sense and rocks all of us to the core, especially when we see how it has devastated his family. Some of his mates fall deeper into drink and drugs, others are shocked out of that way of life. After Tom's funeral, I'm thinking, *Why am I living this way and doing these things? Things have to change.*

Sale are the least 'Danny Cipriani club' in the Premiership. Other clubs were interested, including Bath and Gloucester, but Sale's chief exec Steve Diamond has the gift of the gab and could sell a glass of water to a drowning man.

But I can tell Dimes is genuinely passionate about creating a rugby union stronghold in the north. It's almost as if he's selling a movement. He tells me they're building a formidable pack and how sharp the backline will be, with me added to the likes of Dwayne Peel, Mark Cueto and Sam Tuitupou, all seasoned internationals. Plus, I like the idea of being in a big city like Manchester, where football is king and rugby exists in the shadows. 'Dan,' says Dimes, 'if you want to go out and have a few drinks, you can.' That's nice, because I'm no longer that innocent kid who barely touched a drop.

During pre-season, I realise our pack is nowhere near as formidable as Dimes has made out. Still, I think we're going to be a lot better than we are, which is a shambles. Exeter thump us 43–6 on the first day of the season, we lose our next two games, and forwards coach Steve Scott gets sacked before the end of September. We're booed off after losing to relegation favourites London Welsh at home, and I get dropped to the bench for the next two games. We lose both of those as well. So much for Dimes' northern stronghold, we're the softest touch in the league and the mood around the place is bleak.

Charlie Ingall and I turn up to training one day and Dimes goes mental, tells us we're an hour late. Me and Charlie soon establish that everyone has been told about the change of schedule except us, but Dimes gives us separate dressing downs and we both get written warnings. Afterwards, Charlie tells me that Dimes tried to persuade him to pin the blame on me, so I can't help thinking, *I'm Dimes' marquee signing, I cost a fair few quid, things are going disastrously, is he looking for an excuse to get rid of me already?*

I'm on the bench again for our Heineken Cup game against Cardiff, and we're 15 points down when I'm thrown on with 30 minutes to go. I score our first try, before setting up Mark Jennings for our second. We get another one with five minutes left, the conversion puts us ahead, we win 34–33, and I win man of the match. That proves I've still got it in me to influence games, but how can I start influencing the team, so that we start winning regularly?

It's not like that result turns our season around, we carry on losing most weeks in the Premiership. I can't help remembering what Bryan Redpath said to me during pre-season. 'Fuckin' hell, Danny, our forwards are fuckin' useless. They can't catch or pass. All I can do is tell them to run into contact. What else can I do?'

Those sorts of conversations happen all the time in rugby, it's a coach trying to make a player feel like they have a special bond. We know what's what, even if no-one else does. But I just thought that was Bryan showing a lack of belief in his own ability. Bryan's a lovely fella, and passionate, but I remember thinking, *You're the coach! Don't just tell me how shit my team-mates are, surely it's your job to make them better!* We've got lots of players who are good on paper, we just need a coach with a philosophy, someone who can get us all pulling in the same direction.

We're rock bottom of the league table and staring relegation in the face when Bryan is replaced by former All Blacks coach John Mitchell. The club can't even do that properly. First, reports leak out that Bryan has been sacked, before the club confirm he's been demoted to head coach, Dimes is director of rugby and John is a consultant, whatever that means in practice. I can't help thinking that they suddenly realised they couldn't afford to pay Bryan off.

Our Aussie full-back Cameron Shepherd tells me he was coached by John at Western Force, and that he's absolutely mental. Cam says that during his time at the Force, John concocted some mad, unrealistic drill that involved players running at each other in the gym, over and over again, and resulted in several dislocated knees. John's been around the block and is an imposing presence. Tall, bald as a coot and with different coloured eyes, like David Bowie.

During his first team meeting, he says something along the lines of, 'We're just a bunch of ordinary men trying to do extraordinary things. But if we can be a bunch of extraordinary men trying to do extraordinary things, we're gonna be amazing. And it's one in, all in.'

We beat London Irish, before heading out for a massive team social, on John's orders. I'm all guns blazing, and by the end of the night I'm trying to judo roll John into one of those big food bins you get behind restaurants. Funnily enough, he loves that. But he doesn't love the fact that Richie Gray, our star signing from Scotland, hasn't turned up.

On the Monday, John does this long speech about togetherness and fighting for each other in the trenches, all aimed at Richie. I'm sat there thinking, *This is a bit heavy, just because he didn't come on a piss-up?*

Richie was the club's star signing, a 6 ft 10 in lock with good handling skills and plenty of pace. But if you're a forward with dyed blonde hair and white boots, John and Dimes are coming for you.

John's only at Sale for a couple of months before he walks. No idea why, although Dimes mentions something about him being homesick. I like John, I think he's a unique character, but he hasn't had much of an impact. Since that win over London Irish, we've lost our last three league games.

I've never been in this situation before, fighting tooth and nail for survival. I won the Heineken Cup and Premiership with Wasps, and there was no relegation in Super Rugby, so this is a different kind of pressure entirely. If a couple of things go wrong, you can feel everyone tighten up. I can't play rugby like I want to, because we're not functioning as a team and our only hope is to grind out wins.

Rugby is heavily based on forward dominance – if you've got a dominant pack, the game is a lot more straightforward for the fly-half. But because our pack is usually outgunned or matched, I can't go into a game thinking, *We're going to do this, that and the other*. I've had to work out a different way of playing on the back foot, which means a lot of kicking for territory and rolling mauls, because they're the things we're best at.

I'm constantly assessing, working out a team's weaknesses, making decisions on the hoof. That's great for me, because it means I'm fully engaged in the game, not just passing the ball or kicking, before moving on to the next phase.

It's a seriously steep learning curve and there are plenty of times it feels like I'm slipping back down it. I get hammered in the press after Toulon beat us 62–0 in the Heineken Cup. Our owner even accuses me of not wanting to tackle. He might have a point, but it's not a conscious thing on my part. I don't know for a fact that

Dimes wants me out, but there's certainly that energy in the air. And while I always put my best foot forward for Shaun, I can't put my heart and soul into something if I don't feel I'm being respected.

Since John left, Dimes has put his tracksuit back on and is driving us like slaves. We nick a win against Worcester after Christmas, before managing two in a row against Exeter and London Welsh, which means we're only a point behind London Irish at the bottom of the table. In March, we scrape a one-point win against Bath and draw with Irish. And when we stuff Gloucester and Welsh lose to Northampton in April, Premiership survival is assured.

It's a massive relief, although I don't play a huge part in it. I'm on the bench for most of those run-in games and most people expect me to leave. They're right to think that, because Dimes has told me he'd rather I go. It hasn't been the glorious return home I was hoping for. Then I get hit by a bus.

15

SOME HOPE

There's a load of lads dressed as Oompa Loompas, a few done up as characters from *The Wizard of Oz*, and I'm done up as some WWE wrestler, with my face painted gold and black thunderbolts on my cheeks.

No-one would ever describe me as a conformist, and I still don't drink a huge amount. But when it comes to team socials, I feel like I need to make an effort in order to fit in. Even if it means dressing up like a dickhead and doing the Otley Run, which involves drinking in 15 pubs in and around Leeds, plus the two-hour drive from Manchester. What's the worst that could happen?

I'm drinking rum and cokes and I keep saying to the lads, 'You lot think you're such big men for drinking beer. But this stuff is 40 per cent alcohol.' We've almost made it to the last pub of the crawl and I'm slightly over-excited. I sneak up behind one of the boys, whack him on the back of the head and he starts chasing me. I'm running along, checking over my shoulder, and when I reach a bus stop, I look to my right, see a bus coming, assume it's stopping and make a dash for it. BOOM!

If I hadn't instinctively jumped at the last second and smashed into the bus window instead of the grill, I'd have been wiped out. Legs crushed, maybe killed. As it is, I'm flat on my back on a stretcher, surrounded by paramedics.

As well as being concussed, I've torn the medial collateral ligament in my knee. Not too bad, the season's over anyway. When I get out of hospital, I can't resist tweeting, 'Heavy night. Feel like I've been hit by a bus ...'

People have a laugh at that, which is what I wanted. But no-one asks me how I really am. I suppose it's just par for the course now, me being a fuck up.

Dimes really wants to get rid of me now, and I can't blame him. But something changed that day I got hit by a bus. It's not like I was lying on that stretcher thinking, *My God, this is a life-changing moment*. But I was thinking something along the lines of, *Something really, really has to happen now*.

I'm still taking Tramadol most days, partly for aches and pains, but mostly to numb myself, give me a sense of relief, make me feel cocooned and safe. It also helps me access parts of myself that would otherwise be unreachable.

Tramadol feels like a magic pill. I'll pop one, invite mates over and have deep conversations, with no inhibitions. It's reached a point where I need Tramadol to feel free, but I also know, somewhere deep inside, that I can't be medicating for the rest of my life. Which voice is going to win the battle? The one that promises to make me feel better in the short term, or the one that's telling me I need to actually do some work to feel good naturally?

A week before the bus hit me, my agent James said I should see a guy called Steve Black, who's made his name as Jonny Wilkinson's life coach. I thought, *I've got Shaun, Kevin and Margot to talk to about performance and so on, why do I need someone else?* And I wasn't good at letting new people into my life, so how much could Blackie really do?

But I trust James, he's one of the few people who tells me uncomfortable truths, so I agree to meet Steve in a restaurant in Manchester. I'm not exactly enthusiastic, and I hobble there on crutches like a kid on his way to morning detention. But we end up talking for four hours and I instantly fall in love. No wonder Jonny speaks so highly of this bloke, he's exactly what I needed.

Maybe someone or something was looking down on me, seeing how lost and confused I was, how people were talking about me without knowing me at all, how little I knew myself. Maybe it saw all the mistakes I kept making, how I looked like an obstinate ram, banging my head against a brick wall, backing up and doing it again, because I didn't know I had the capacity to do any different. Maybe it saw all this and said, 'This kid needs to stop wasting his talent, blaming everyone else and start taking care of himself. Tell you what I'm gonna do, get a bus to almost kill him before sending him to Blackie.'

Blackie's wisdom doesn't come from books – although he is well-read – it comes from real life, and it comes from the heart. In olden times, he probably would have been a village sage. He tells me about his past life as a bouncer in Newcastle, how he knocked out the wrong guy, almost killed him and had to go on the run, because the local mob were on his tail.

Blackie tried to be a boxer for a bit, until he realised throwing punches in the ring is very different to throwing punches on the street. That's when he started figuring out who he was and what he could be, which is the kind, gentle, generous, joyful, all-round wonderful human being he is now.

Now me and Blackie are meeting once a week. Sometimes he comes down to me, sometimes I head up to Newcastle. Every time he walks into the room, it lights up. And in between our meetings, we're chatting on the phone all the time. Even then I can feel his energy pulsing down the line.

Counselling works wonders for a lot of people, but I feel talked down to by psychotherapists. It's very prescriptive, with techniques and rules. I've been finding my own way since I was a kid, so for me it's about feel. Blackie's with me in the trenches, and we're going to get through things together.

I've had coaches, like Shaun and Brian, who knew me well, but they only knew as much as I gave them. You have to allow someone to open the bonnet and see your inner workings for them to get to know you intimately.

Every time I speak to Blackie, there are at least three lightbulb moments. Probably because he has a chequered past, and been wrongly judged because of it, he cuts through all the bullshit he's heard about me, sees me for who I really am and speaks to that person. He helps me figure out a lot of the thoughts that are swirling around my head, makes me feel cared for and loved, in a way I imagine a father cares for and loves his son. I've been in a lonely place for a long time, but now I've met this amazing man, I've got some hope to cling to.

Blackie's intuitive, understands that an athlete's character will dictate how he plays his sport. He understands that quirks can be a positive, if harnessed properly. And because he's a normal bloke, whose wisdom comes from experience and how he's felt, he understands that advice is best served without frills. Like he says, 'Life is simple, we just make it complicated.'

Blackie writes me little notes, things to do with performance and diet, or to help me get my thoughts back on track if they're going wayward. If other people saw them, they might wonder what the fuss was about. But it's precisely because they're so simple, and flow so easily, that they work. He also gets me writing a performance journal, in which I meticulously record everything I eat, what I do and don't do well in training, and how I feel mentally.

After a few weeks working with Blackie, I say to Dimes, 'I'm sorting myself out. When I come back for pre-season, I'll be ready.'

Sure enough, when pre-season comes, I feel better than I've ever felt on a rugby field. Not only am I 100 per cent engaged in every session, but I'm also trying to make sure everyone else is. I'll say to the younger lads, 'How do you think we should do this? Maybe we should do it like this instead?' I want to make them think differently about areas of the game they thought they knew.

What Bryan said to me last season, about the forwards being useless and not being able to improve their skills, has stayed with me. It's not like I thought, *I'm gonna teach everyone how to play rugby properly*. But I have realised that if I don't do it, none of the coaches will. Upskilling my team-mates will make my job easier and produce better results for the team.

I'm back with Kelly. And my God has it been a drawn-out process. I felt like something was missing and convinced myself she'd be the answer to all my problems. But after a couple of weeks, I realised I'd made a terrible mistake.

What I felt for Kelly wasn't real love. It can't have been, because now she's back, I still feel lonely and lacking, with a big hole that hasn't been filled. And that pain I felt without her wasn't longing, it was my ego being crushed.

We chug along for months, until one day, this PR guy says to me that someone close to me was leaking my whereabouts to the paparazzi. After that, my trust in those closest to me was broken, including Kelly, although I'm not saying she was responsible, in fact I don't know who it was. At that point, in my head it felt like the relationship was over.

I've never spoken to the media about any of my relationships, whereas I've had countless women speak about me. For some of them, their whole existence revolved around getting as much attention as possible. Being photographed with me all the time was great for their careers, because it kept their names in the media.

It's a thrill the first few times you leave a venue, the photographers are clamouring and flashes are going off all around you. But after a while, that kind of attention is hell, at least for most people. You feel like an exotic fish in an aquarium, with people looking in, their noses pressed against the glass.

That's why celebrities usually hang out with other celebrities, because only they can understand how it feels to be seen as not fully human. And it's probably the only thing me and Kelly actually have in common.

I never wanted to be part of a celebrity package, a couple that creates a furore whenever they go out for dinner. And I would have swapped all that attention for people to know the truth. Then again, I'm still figuring out who I am, because I'm still being dictated to, by people I don't even know.

I slip into my old ways, messaging women with wild abandon. And it doesn't take long for Kelly to rumble me. She goes through my phone, sees all these conversations I've been having, some of them pretty X-rated, and calls quite a few of the numbers. She tells me it's over, boots me out of her house and the press get wind of the story in no time. Now, on top of everything else, I'm a love rat and an out-of-control sex maniac. And, for once, it's accurate.

Just as it felt like I was getting a grip on one part of my life, namely my rugby, other parts are getting away from me. Blackie is sifting through the clutter of my mind, but it's still a bit of a mess. These things, he tells me, don't happen overnight.

16

TWEAKING AND IMPROVING

I was complacent during my first season with Sale. I'd expected to return from Australia and for it all to go swimmingly. I'd allowed myself to be at the mercy of my coaches and how they saw the game. I wasn't going to allow that to happen again.

The club expected me to come straight into this new environment and perform miracles. But that doesn't happen by chance. You have to treat a player right, make him feel wanted, part of the group. Instead, as soon as it went tits up, which was pretty much from the start, they wanted me out.

I'd wear the 'wrong' kit at training, which I didn't think was important, but which drove some people mad. They'd think it was a sign of laziness and/or disrespect, or that I didn't see myself as part of the team. Maybe there was something going on in my subconscious mind, that I saw wearing the 'wrong' kit as striking a blow against conformity. Then again, Shaun wore the 'wrong' kit all the time, and he's the best coach I've worked with.

I lived in Manchester city centre that first season and was late for training a few times, which isn't ideal, especially if you're the fly-half. But with Dimes, it would be like the end of the world. 'What the fuck do you think you're doing?! Fucking get over here and explain yourself!' I'd be thinking, *Come on, man, the traffic was bad. There's nothing I could do. It's not like I feel good about it, can't we just crack on and have a good session?* At Wasps people were late all the time, and we won far more than we lost.

But that first season with Sale was a valuable learning experience. I no longer want to be at the mercy of a coach's system or philosophy that doesn't feel right, because the one thing I do trust about myself is my feel for the game.

Everything I do with Blackie is about taking responsibility, and one of the key responsibilities of a fly-half is running the show. At Wasps, I was lucky to have lots of great players around me. But at Sale, I need to understand everyone else's role. And if I'm allowed to run a system, I can make sure all the right people are in all the right places, and control results to a certain extent.

I feel like a different player at the start of the 2013–14 season. And I'm confident enough to say to Dimes, 'Look, this is what's happening this season. This is what we need to do.' That said, I'm not even in the squad for our first two league games, he has me playing for the reserves instead.

As well as the work I've been doing with Blackie, I've been training with Margot all summer. I'm fit as a fiddle and my mind feels razor-sharp. If Dimes isn't outright taking the piss out of me, he's certainly playing some sort of game. I'm angry and frustrated, but Blackie tells me not to worry, that it's a long season and things will change if I just keep doing what I'm doing.

People think professional athletes will naturally bring the right attitude to every training session, but it's easy to drift when they're not particularly inspiring. But Blackie has me firing on all cylinders every single session. If the coaches aren't going to make it inspiring for everyone, I will. I'm not intense and frantic, I'm just 100 per cent tuned in. And because other players, especially the young ones, are tuning into my frequency, it's benefiting the whole team.

I'm on the bench for the game against Wasps and only get on after Nick Macleod gets injured halfway through the first half. But I play the house down, scoring a try, setting another one up and kicking 16 points in a 26–22 win.

Suddenly, Dimes is my best mate, and he even comes out for drinks with me, Mark Cueto and some other lads. But I still remember his disdain, and I get the feeling he's only keeping me close now I've become more useful to him.

I didn't watch much of the 2011 World Cup, but I can't say I was surprised at how poorly we performed, because Martin Johnson's coaching team was like most coaching teams in English rugby, based on a mixture of fear, stats and rigid structure.

The aim of rugby is to attack space, at least it should be. If you're always running straight at defenders, without much nuance, you're relying too heavily on your physicality. The top international sides are fairly evenly matched physically, so it's game intelligence and execution of skills that will set you apart.

If the RFU could have created an England head coach in a laboratory, he would have been a lot like Stuart Lancaster. Lanny looks the right way, says the right things, loves his country and comes across as very thoughtful. Meet the new boss, same as the old boss – except this one is expected to keep his troops in check.

Lanny and I have a bit of a rocky history, so on a personal level, his appointment is something of a disaster. Before a Saxons game against Italy A in 2010, Lanny wanted us to do a drop-goal routine in training. I thought, *We're playing Italy's second team, for fuck's sake. You only kick a drop-goal to win a game in the dying seconds. If we haven't put four or five tries past them before then, something's gone horribly wrong*. When the ball came back to me, instead of kicking a drop-goal, I hit a cross-field ball and the winger scored in the corner.

Lanny was shouting, 'No! No! No! We need you to kick a drop-goal!' But I was feeling a bit defiant now, so when the ball came to me a second time, I stepped outside, threw a miss pass, and the winger scored in the other corner.

Lanny's head went purple, looked like it was going to explode. He used to be a teacher, so I imagine he hated not being in control. But I wasn't doing something pointless just because he told me to, I was doing what I felt was right, for me and the team.

After the 2013 autumn internationals, it's same old, same old in the media. Not enough inspiration, not enough intuition, not enough creativity. It's been like a broken record since we won the World Cup in 2003. Meanwhile, I'm playing some great rugby for Sale, so it's hardly surprising that journalists and pundits are saying I should be back in the England fold.

Toby Flood's decided to join Toulouse, which has probably ended his international career, but Lanny picks Saracens' Owen Farrell and Bath's George Ford for his 2014 Six Nations training camp, while I'm not even in the Saxons squad. England have a decent Six Nations, finishing second behind Ireland, but the clamour to include me in the squad for the New Zealand tour is building.

On paper, Sale's team isn't as good as the previous season, but we're squeezing every drop from what we've got. The young guys, like Sam James, Mike Haley and Will Addison, are buying into the ideas I'm sharing with them, and I'm getting all their youthful energy and excitement in return.

I've also got a scrum-half in Dwayne Peel who knows his principle role is to pass me the ball as quickly as possible. Dwayne loves running, and because he's a Welsh international I back him to do his thing more than I would other nines. But if he runs and it doesn't come off, I'll get stuck into him. That's just poor decision-making, running because it might catch the eye, rather than because it's best for the team. I'll say to Dwayne, 'Your one job is to give me the ball', and while I say it in a joking tone, just to mess with him, I mean it.

I've never been the same running threat since I injured my ankle, certainly don't make as many eye-catching breaks as I did in my first couple of years with Wasps. But there's a spring back in my step, and I'm a more complete player these days, more focused on getting everyone around me ticking.

Annoyingly, the England coaches see me running laterally and think it's a weakness. What they don't realise is I'm running laterally to draw defenders towards me, which creates space for my two massive centres, whose strength is running straight and hard. Or maybe they do realise, and they need another excuse not to pick me.

They can't keep accusing me of being iffy defensively, because I'm near the top of the tackling stats with Sale. Then again, that doesn't stop people writing articles accusing me of shirking my defensive responsibilities, including Stuart Barnes, who describes me as a 'speed bump' after a game against Worcester.

Stuart was a creative fly-half who didn't win many caps for England, which is probably why he normally writes these things about me. But I feel moved to get in touch with him and explain the modern realities of defence.

What looks like a missed tackle, and will be recorded as such, is often a fly-half rushing up fast to force the attacker infield. And a lot of my tackling is hitting people high, because I know that someone else will finish them off low. That way, I remain on my feet in the defensive line, rather than stuck at the bottom of a ruck.

* * *

We beat league leaders Northampton in March, comfortably, and I get Premiership player of the month. A couple of games later, we put 50 points on Exeter to secure a top-six finish and a place in the Champions Cup, as the Heineken Cup has been rebranded. A few weeks later, I'm named in the England squad for the tour of New Zealand.

Owen Farrell can't do the first Test, because he's playing for Saracens in the Premiership final, as is Northampton's Stephen Myler, while George Ford is injured. Had they all been available, there's no way I'd have gone. As it is, Gloucester's Freddie Burns, the other fly-half in the squad for the first Test, has had an ordinary season, by his own admission, so I'm thinking, *Surely I'm starting?*

When I was in Martin Johnson's squad, I mistakenly thought I'd be allowed to speak my mind and at least be heard, like at Wasps. But it's a case of keeping my head down and letting my training do the talking.

We've got so many players unavailable for the first Test in Auckland and no-one's beaten the All Blacks at Eden Park for 20 years, so everyone expects us to get battered. They pick Freddie to start, with me on the bench, apparently because Freddie did well as a replacement when they beat the All Blacks in 2012.

We're losing 15–12 when I come on with nine minutes left. I make a line break and win a penalty, which I kick from 40 metres out, and suddenly Eden Park is deathly silent. But with three minutes to go, Conrad Smith goes over in the corner to clinch the win for New Zealand.

The cavalry returns for the second Test defeat in Dunedin, while I'm not even in the squad. But Owen is injured for the third Test in Hamilton, so Freddie starts and I'm on the bench again, despite playing well in a big midweek win over the Crusaders, which is my first England start for six years.

New Zealand score four tries before the break and we're not at the races. It's so poor, I think I'll be going on after half-time, but I don't get on straight after the break and we end up losing 36–13. Having looked decent in the first Test, with a bunch of unsung players in the team, we suddenly look miles away from being World Cup contenders in 2015. But on a personal level, I thought I'd looked at home back on the international stage.

Paul Deacon has joined Sale from rugby league and we've really clicked. The reason league guys are often successful when they switch to coaching union is partly down to the fact that they're down to earth, working-class lads with humility. But it's also because rugby league is so much more structured.

Rugby league has the six-tackle rule, no line-outs, no mauls and no proper rucks or scrums. An attacking player is expected to keep the ball in the tackle, so defences are usually very well-organised, which means in order to break a defence down, you have to get your shapes of attack just right. Consequently, top league players know all about running lines, tempo and timing, fixing and manipulating defenders, drawing and passing.

Deac brings new perspectives and lots of detail but is also hungry to learn. We talk about rugby for ages – the way he sees and feels about things, the way I see and feel about things. Sometimes he'll think a league pattern will do a job in union and I'll be sceptical, because union and league defences are so different. He'll insist I try it a few times anyway, and if it doesn't, we'll sit down and find a way to make it work. It's a two-way relationship, and I can see the improvements he's making, to my game and the rest of the team's.

Deac brings a new attacking system, which I love, but we've tweaked and improved it. Unlike other coaches, he's receptive to my point of view, so we're like a couple of old mates under a car bonnet, fine-tuning an engine.

In our system, the forwards know exactly where they've got to be, and there is an emphasis on the forwards executing plays, whether it be making a two-yard pass or playing out the back, while another wave of forwards hits the line. As for the backs, they always provide options, whether on the short side or behind the forwards' running lines.

At one team meeting, Deac shows a clip of me kicking a long punt deep into the other team's half. Then he says, 'You kicked the ball away, maybe you should have kept the ball in hand.' Silence. I have to say something. 'But Deac, sometimes you have to kick for territory, to relieve the pressure and attack from inside their half.' Afterwards, Dimes takes Charlie Ingall aside and says, 'Everyone else just agrees with things, why does Danny always have to be disruptive?'

That's the difference between a coach from a rugby league background and a dyed in the wool union man. While league is a proudly working-class sport, union is overwhelmingly middle-class. And the middle-classes tend to be more conformist, because their lives tend to be more structured. Generally speaking, middle-class kids have parents with respectable jobs, live in nice houses, go to nice schools. They're inculcated with the idea that people in charge – parents, teachers, coaches – know best, and only if you do as they say will you progress. And they carry that attitude into adulthood, so that when they become parents, teachers or coaches, they think they know best, too.

In contrast, there are studies which appear to show that kids who grow up in less structured environments, with less parental guidance, make more of their own decisions. In some cases, they're having to make their own decisions simply to get through the day safely. As a result, they grow up with more elastic minds than middle-class kids, and are more likely to have a looser, more exuberant approach to sport. I also reckon they're less likely to assume that someone knows better simply because they're in a position of authority.

The problem is, when you're plucked out of that world and placed in a structured environment, you're going to stick out like a sore thumb. You're wanting to stretch your mind and run free, while almost all your peers are in lockstep, craving conformity and comfort. Meanwhile, your coaches are wanting to rein you in and batter you back into an 'acceptable' shape.

Playing rugby should involve making constant decisions in the moment – making the right pass, running the right support line – but if you're coached rigidly, you'll play rigidly. If you're thinking about what your coaches want you to do, rather than thinking for yourself, you'll play in a staccato fashion, rather than with fluidity. You'll almost always take the safe option, instead of what might be the right one.

I don't know much about Dimes' background, but he's been in that stifling rugby union environment for a long time. So instead of thinking, *Danny's been doing this for years now, he knows what works and what doesn't, best to take a step back and let him and the rest of the boys get on with it*, he has that old-school mindset of, *Do as the coach says, end of story.*

MARK CUETO

When Cips arrived on the scene with England, his skill was off the charts. He was doing stuff with a rugby ball that even Dan Carter could only dream of.

But rather than embracing and promoting this rare talent, as would have happened in football, a negative narrative soon grew up around Cips: *he doesn't respect rugby's traditions, he's getting too big for his boots, he's more interested in being a celebrity.*

Cips made mistakes, but maybe he'd have made fewer if someone he respected in the England set-up had put their arm around him and said, 'You're in the public domain now, you've got to be more careful.' What happened instead? While one of the most naturally gifted fly-halves in the world was being criticised and ostracised, England fans kept asking why their team wasn't very exciting. Talk about cutting off your nose to spite your face.

One of the biggest problems with rugby is that if a player gets a negative label slapped on him early in his career, it's almost impossible to lose it.

One of my best mates is Charlie Hodgson, who I played with for 10 years at Sale. In the early days, Charlie's defence wasn't great. Not terrible, just nowhere near as good as Jonny Wilkinson's. As time went on, it got a lot better, to the point that it was unusual for him to miss a tackle. But he never stopped being labelled as poor defensively, just as Cips never stopped being labelled as poor defensively, which hampered both their England careers.

But Cips wasn't just unfairly judged for his actions on the field, he was also unfairly judged for his off-field activities. When David Beckham started dating a Spice Girl, it was just the natural way of things, all part of the glitz and glamour of football, a great way of taking the game to a wider audience. But when Cips went out with beautiful celebrities, he got crucified: 'Who the hell does he think he is?' Meanwhile, people in rugby were scratching their heads and asking, 'How do we grow the game?'

Sadly, not much seems to have changed. When Maro Itoje was photographed with Jay-Z a couple of years back, it should have been seen as a positive thing, an English rugby player hobnobbing with one of the biggest music artists on the planet. Instead, people were telling Maro to concentrate on his rugby.

I must admit, I wasn't a big fan of Cips in his early days, probably because I was caught up in the idea that there was a hierarchy that needed to be respected and rugby wasn't a sport for superstars. But when I found out that Cips was coming to

Sale, I was excited, because I'd seen how good he was with Wasps, and in that game for England against Ireland in 2008.

When you bring a marquee player into a club, you want them to raise standards. And that's exactly what Cips did. He had so much knowledge and passion and wanted everything to be perfect. At times, it was like having the head coach playing alongside you. It was like he was playing chess, moving people exactly where he wanted them to be on the field. That kind of attention to detail, bordering on obsession, is great. But it can rub people up the wrong way.

Usually when someone plays poorly, they'll keep their head down the following week. But with Cips, it didn't make any difference. He'd be chirping away in training as normal, telling everyone what to do. I know some guys would be thinking, *Concentrate on your own fucking job*. Sometimes they'd even say it. But Cips got better at communicating his ideas as he matured, and he got on well with all his team-mates. As for me, I loved him to bits.

Saying I was like a father figure to Cips would be too strong – I'm not that old – but I certainly felt like an older brother. I recently bumped into him at Twickenham, the day France hammered England 53–10. I hadn't spoken to him for months, but we gave each other a big hug and he was chatting away to my missus and kids like he really was my kid brother.

That's the obvious point that most people miss about Cips: rugby teams are close-knit, so you have to be a decent lad to be accepted. If Cips had been the knobhead the media made him out to be, Sale would have turfed him out in no time, because his team-mates wouldn't have played for him. Instead, people could see that his heart was in the right place, and that he sometimes got things wrong only because he was so driven. And it's because he was so driven that he managed to get Sale ticking, as he did every team he played for.

Cips was that rare combination of exceptional natural talent and relentless work ethic, so I can only think that successive England coaches didn't fancy him because they were influenced by what was being written and said about him. I can see why an England coach would pick Owen Farrell ahead of Cips, just as I can see why they'd pick Owen over Marcus Smith today. But Cips should have been more involved, no doubt about that.

And it goes deeper than what Cips could have done for England on the pitch. I worry about rugby, there's so much negativity surrounding it. If I'm not reading a story about another player with a brain injury, I'm reading a story about another club going bust. Rugby is never going to compete with football, in terms of viewership or finances, but there's enough interest out there for it to be sustainable. But to be sustainable, it's got to make the most of any stars in its ranks, instead of tearing them down, like it did with Cips.

17

THE ONLY THING I EVER WANTED

On paper, our squad should be battling relegation, but Sale continue to over-perform in the 2014–15 season because we've found ways of winning games when we're physically outmatched.

We're very good at pinpointing a team's weak links. We know we can't just give the ball to a big guy, expect him to get over the gain line and launch an attack from there. We have to go out the back, use short passes and different angles instead. Not that Lanny is impressed, because I'm not in the England squad for the autumn internationals. Am I surprised? Not really. Disappointed? Yeah, a bit. But don't worry about me, I'll dust myself down and go again, like I always do.

I read it all the time in the papers, variations on 'Farrell/Ford/Myler wins personal duel with Cipriani.' What they neglect to mention is that those three guys are playing behind formidable packs and on the front foot most weeks. Some guys get it, and Worcester head coach Dean Ryan says it best in his newspaper column: 'It's the number 10 who keeps his head, his eye for a gap, a mismatch or an overlap in extremis, who is the better Test match decision-maker.'

People are always saying, 'Test rugby is different to club rugby.' It is, but not in the way most people think. Playing for England is easier than playing for your club, because you're surrounded by the best talent in the country, people who are as motivated as you and more attuned to what you're doing. Look at what happened against Ireland in 2008, the only time I was allowed to run the attack for England – it was a walk in the park.

That said, if you've spent your entire club career playing behind a dominant pack, you're going to struggle when you're playing for England and your pack only has parity or a slight edge, because you've never had to work out how to play on the back foot.

Owen, George and Stephen are obviously very good players with their own strengths, but it's frustrating to be continuously overlooked for three guys with a similar skillset. I can only imagine my reputation precedes me, that the coaches are worried I'll say too much, or too many of the wrong things. It seems to be okay for others to make their voices heard, but I guess they're saying what the coaches want to hear.

England are beaten by New Zealand and South Africa at Twickenham, which makes it five losses in a row. So now people are starting to panic. 'ENGLAND DESPERATELY NEED MORE CREATIVITY,' says the *Guardian*, 'ENGLAND DO NOT HAVE ENOUGH PLAYMAKERS,' says the *Times*, 'ENGLAND LACK INTELLIGENCE,' says the *Observer*, 'ENGLAND HAVE NO X-FACTOR,' says the *Mirror*. 'ENGLAND ARE CRYING OUT FOR MAVERICKS,' says the *Telegraph*.

Truth be told, I'm ambivalent about the 'maverick' descriptor, because it has negative connotations. It suggests I'm flash, flaky, a liability, a luxury, a risk, an individual in a team game. It suggests I do unorthodox things for the sake of it, to entertain people, just for the craic. But that's not true. I just see the game differently to most, probably because I didn't grow up with people drilling me how to play it.

When I was a kid, it was only ever about attacking space and doing the right thing in the moment. Playing the game that way gave me so much joy – and success – that I never thought about playing it differently as an adult. But an awful lot of work goes into it. I spend hundreds of hours honing my skillset, building a deep trust in myself, so that I'm able to follow my impulses. As Blackie says, 'You've got your box of tricks, it's about pulling the right one out at the right time.'

We have a culture in England of sportspeople not being allowed to express themselves, on and off the field. And I play a sport that epitomises that. Rugby union in England is staid and constrictive, suspicious of difference. Because I come from a different place and have a different perspective, they don't know how to handle me. So they stick a label on me, which marks me as the problem.

When sportspeople can't express themselves, be who they really want, they can't fulfil their potential. How many truly pioneering rugby union players has England produced in the professional era? Not many.

It's true that when I was a kid, I tried things that weren't on. But Shaun got on my back about that. And as time went on, I looked deeper and deeper, discovered how things work, improved my decision-making and learned how to get a grip of a team. And when I do make mistakes, they're quickly consigned to the past.

Anyone who watches me play often will know that I'm essentially a traditional fly-half now. But I'm technically far better and a lot more nuanced than I used to be. I'm also consistent, delivering performances almost every week. As for the disruptive tag, anyone who's played with me will tell you I'm nothing of the sort. I'm a team man, desperate for everyone at Sale to be successful. It's just that some coaches are afraid of having conversations, which frustrates me, and sometimes makes me look like a bit of a malcontent.

Lanny's in the stands when I score a try and set up another in a win over Exeter, and he's there again when we upset league leaders Northampton. Toulon want to sign me as a replacement for Jonny Wilkinson, who's retiring. But that would scupper my England hopes, and playing for England is still the be all and end all as far as my rugby ambitions are concerned.

Lanny can't keep ignoring me, not if I keep playing like this, so I'm staying put.

* * *

Having Blackie in my corner gives me hope. He's even trying to build a relationship with Lanny, so that maybe he'll understand me better.

I don't know what Blackie's saying to him, probably stuff along the lines of, 'Just get to know him, find out what he's really about, look how much he's improved since he's been working with me.' Whatever it is, I respect Lanny for being willing to listen. But Blackie also relays some of the things Lanny's been telling him, which aren't encouraging.

Lanny already had a negative opinion of me, partly because of when he coached me with the Saxons, partly because of the things he'd heard. He's a good person, just very strait-laced, the kind of guy who's always got his trainers tied up tight, his polo shirt tucked neatly into his shorts and his hair a sensible length. Everything about him seems measured and in order, and he has taught me a few things about stability, consistency and being accountable.

But I'm not too surprised when Blackie tells me that people I thought were friends have been getting in Lanny's ear, telling him I'm not to be trusted. And because it confirms what Lanny already believes, as well as solving a potentially thorny problem, he's leaning towards believing them.

Blackie gets more and more frustrated at how they're treating me, how they're unwilling to even try to fit me in. He never says anything rude to Lanny, but he says to me, 'Danny, be careful who you speak to and what you say, because no-one is fighting your corner in that camp.'

I'm in England's 2015 Six Nations training squad, at least for the first game against Wales, so I tell Dimes I'll be at Sale next season, rather than moving to France. Then Owen suffers a bad knee injury and is ruled out for the tournament, which means they can't really discard me.

Lanny's assistant Andy Farrell is the man in charge of England. I get on well with Andy, we can have a laugh and a joke. He's a very good coach, with lots of insight he's brought from league. I like the way he wants England to play, with a bit of devil, and he gives me some great advice about foot speed and tempo. But I start on the bench in Cardiff and remain there for the next 80 minutes. We win and George Ford plays well, but it's tough not to get a run-out.

Against Italy, I come on with 18 minutes to go. I'm afraid of how the crowd will react, because I'm convinced everyone hates me. If you read it enough, you start to believe it. But there's a big cheer and I start to well up. *These people actually want me in the team. Jeez, this is overwhelming ...*

I score with my first touch, but don't celebrate. Instead, I'm thinking, *Don't even smile, Lanny might think you're gloating.*

Between the Italy win and the potential Grand Slam decider against Ireland, I'm in the Sale team that beats Saracens. Some win that is. But I'm on the bench in Dublin, and what's happening now makes no sense at all.

We're 10 points down with 22 minutes to go, George is having a rough time of it, and we haven't even looked like scoring a try. They chuck on five replacements – a new hooker, a new prop, a new number eight, a new scrum-

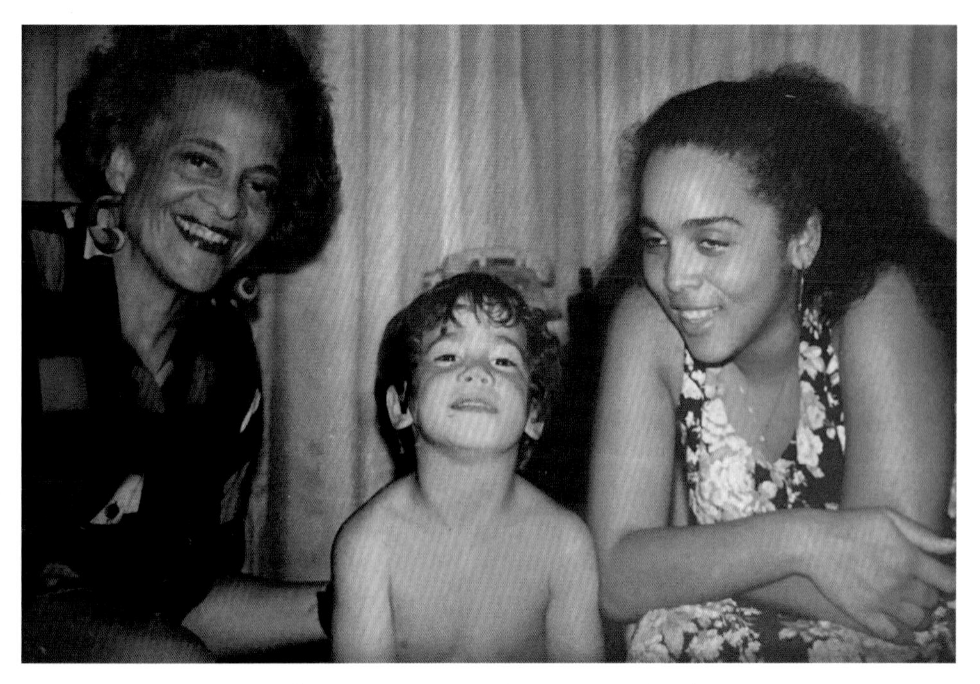

With Auntie Rosie and my cousin Trisha.

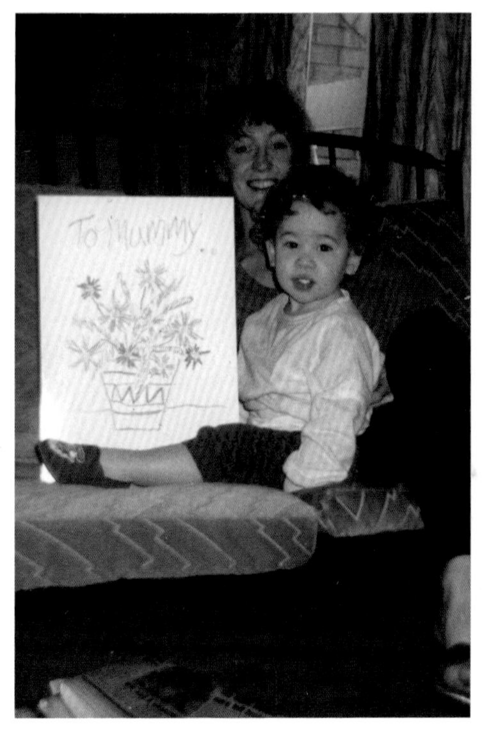

An early photo
with Mum.

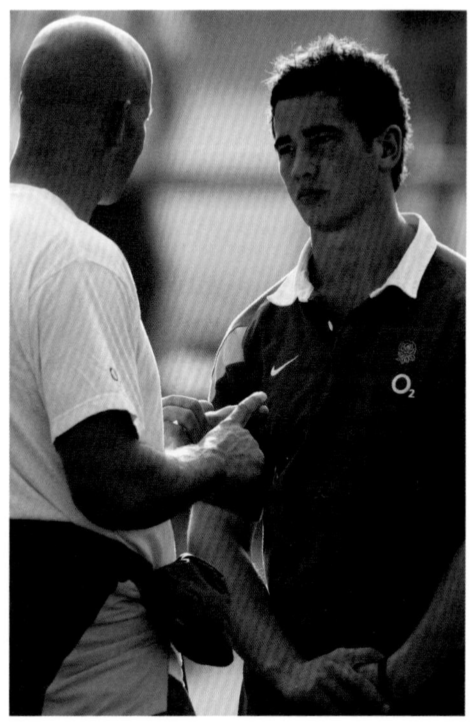

England camp, 2006. I always
listened to my coaches. I didn't
always agree with them.

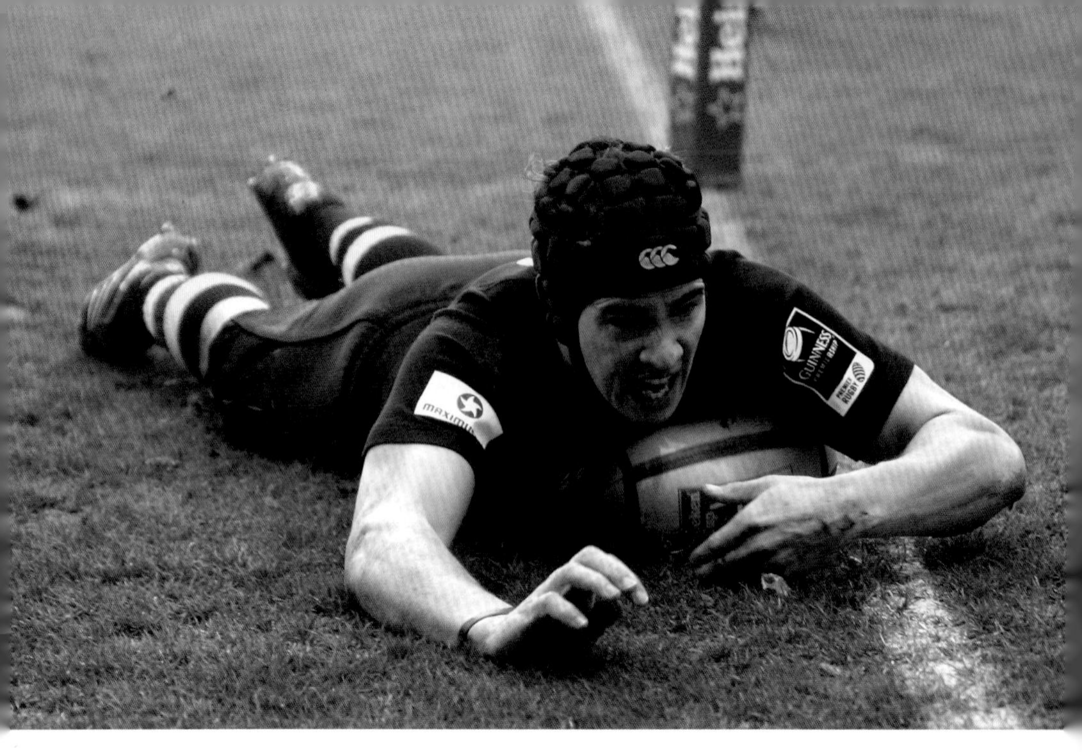

Try-time for Wasps against Leinster in the Heineken Cup, 2007.

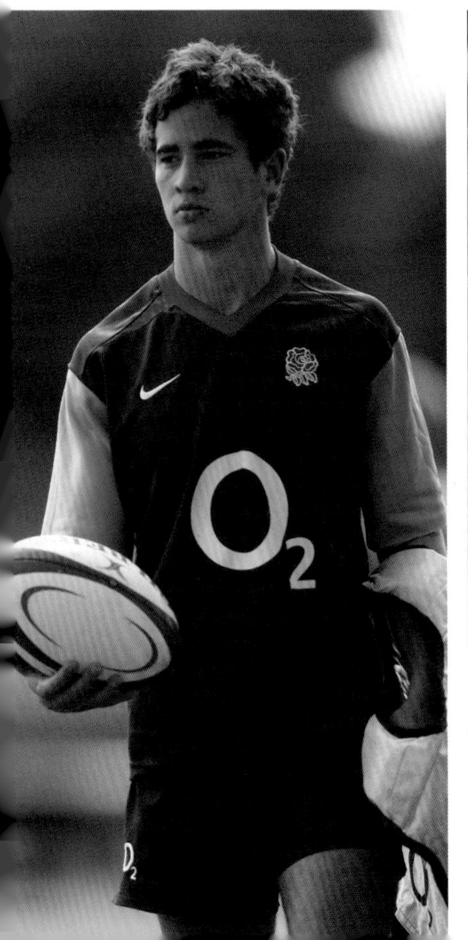

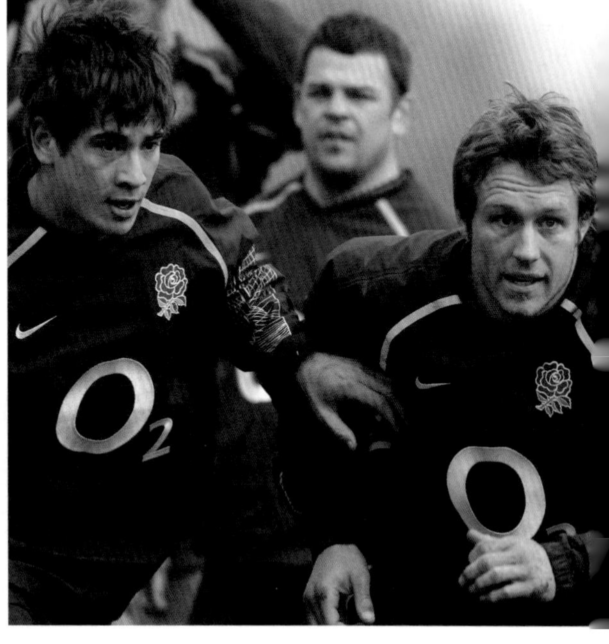

Above: Contrary to media reports, Jonny Wilkinson and I loved playing and competing together.

Left: Training with England in 2007.

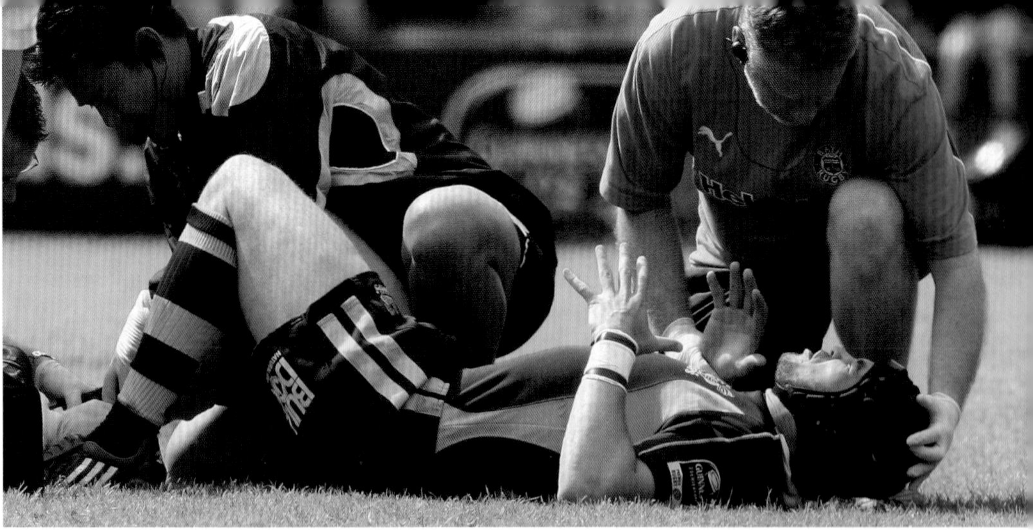

Above: Injuries are a part of sport, but my leg injury in 2008 was devastating.

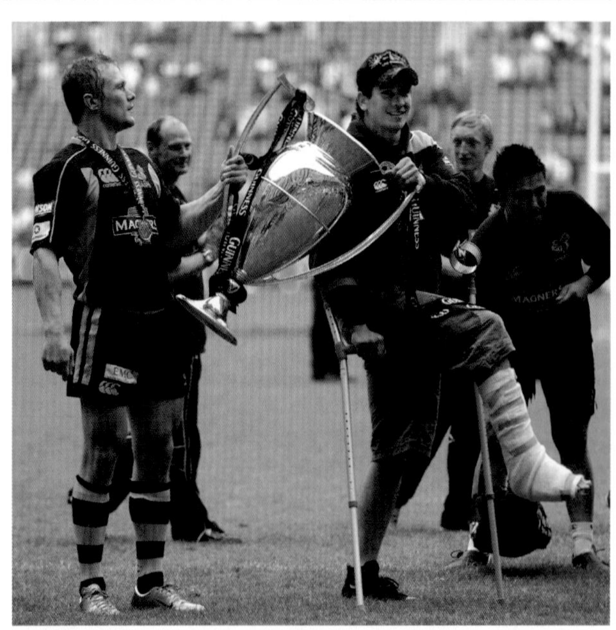

Right: Celebrating beating Leicester in the Premiership final at Twickenham, 2008.

Below: Playing for Brian Ashton always brought out the best in me.

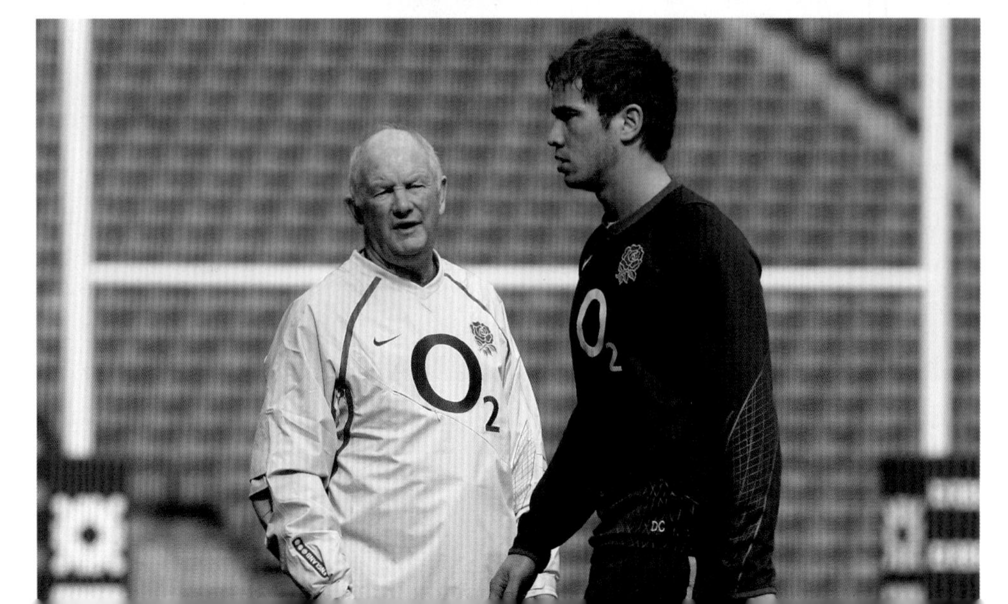

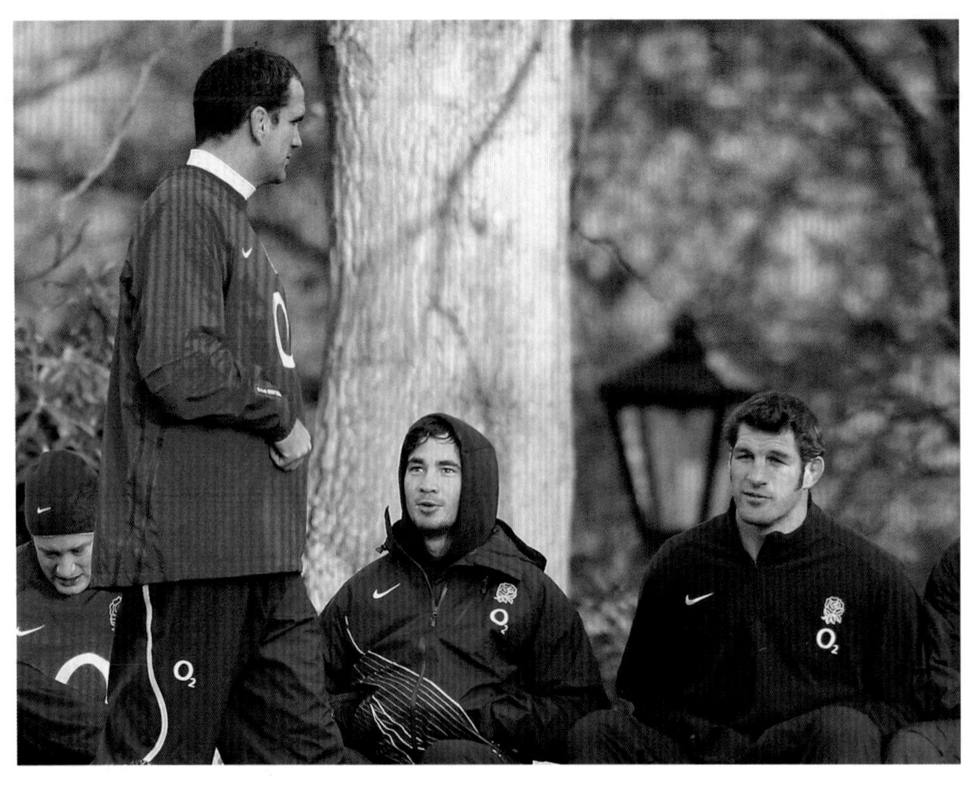

Martin Johnson holding court at training with England.

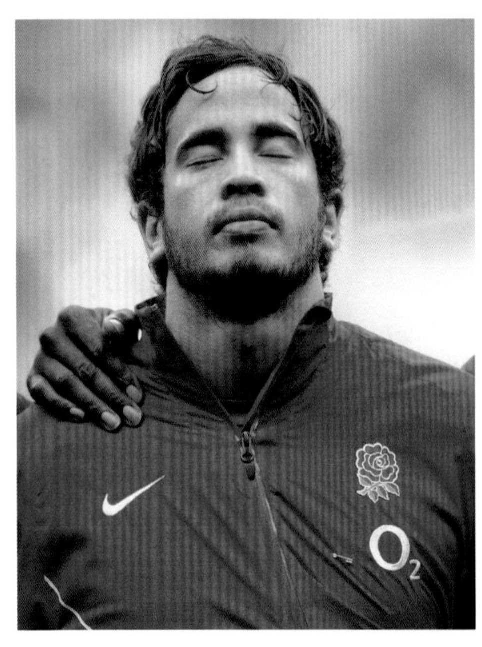

Playing for England in 2008. There is no better feeling than hearing the national anthem.

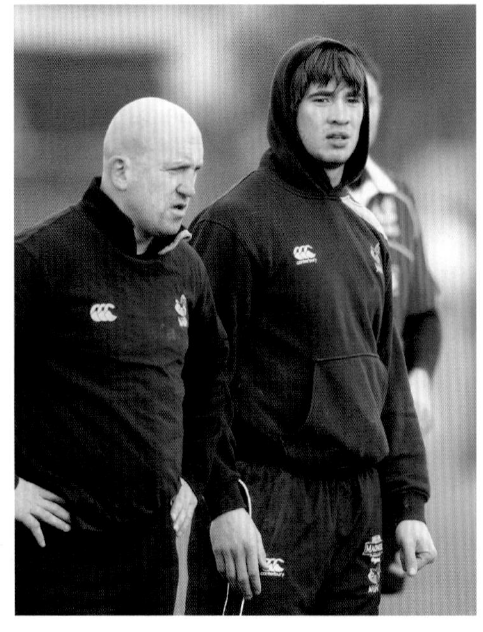

I loved playing for Shaun Edwards: a truly great coach and mentor.

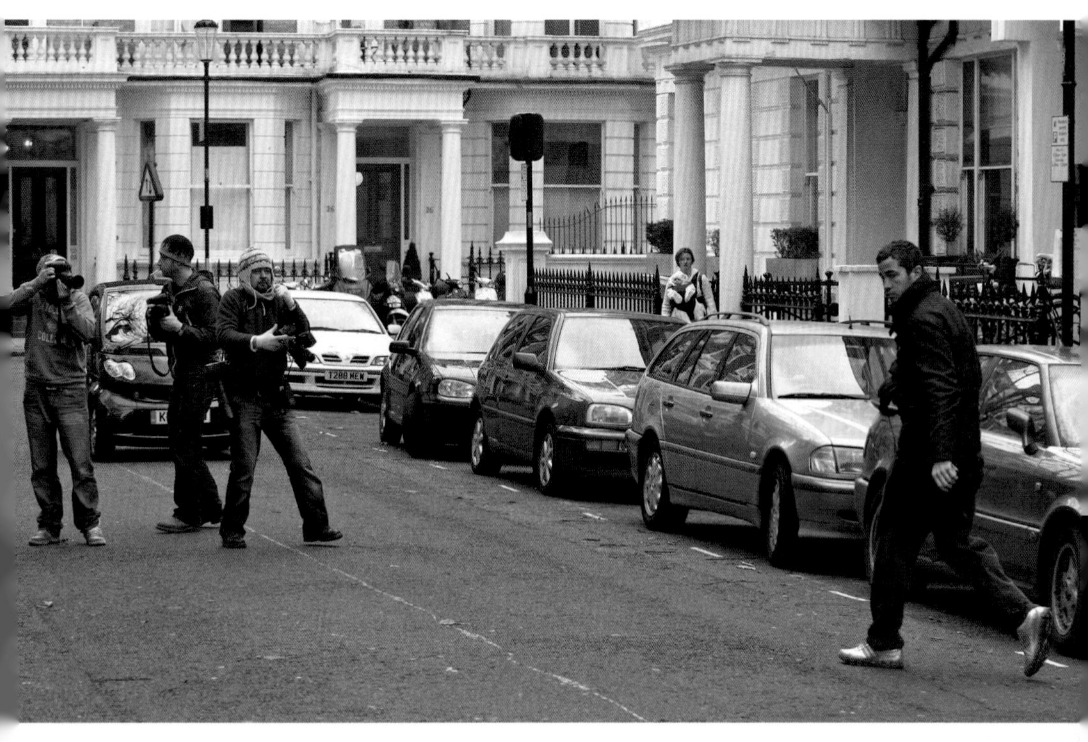

Getting papped on the streets where I lived was a regular occurrence.

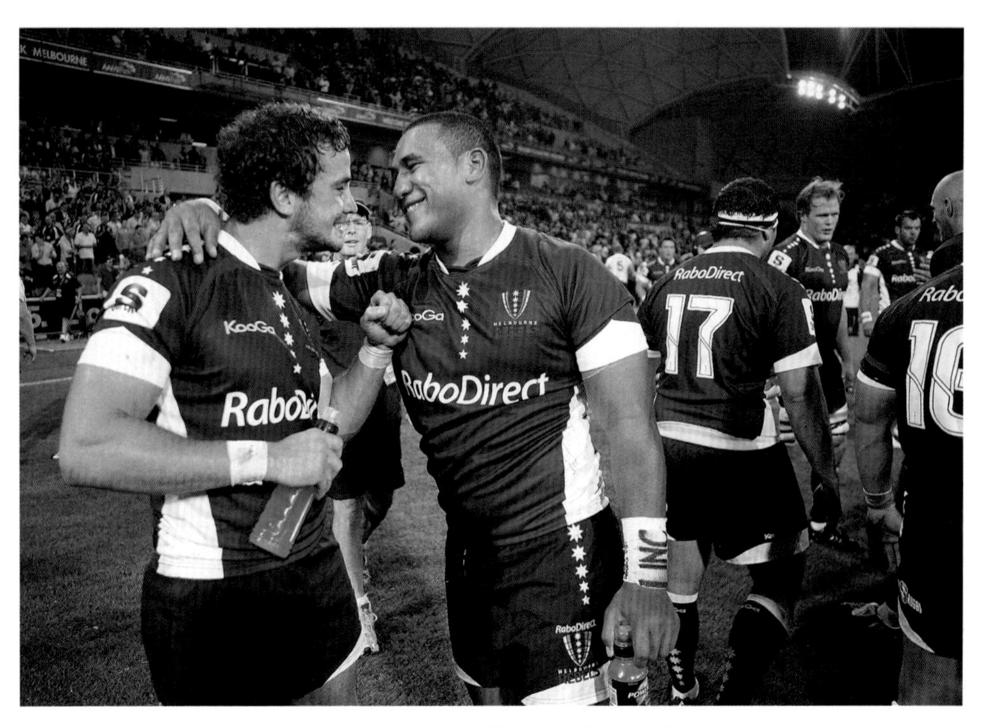

My time in Australia was short and not always sweet,
but I learned a lot about myself and my game.

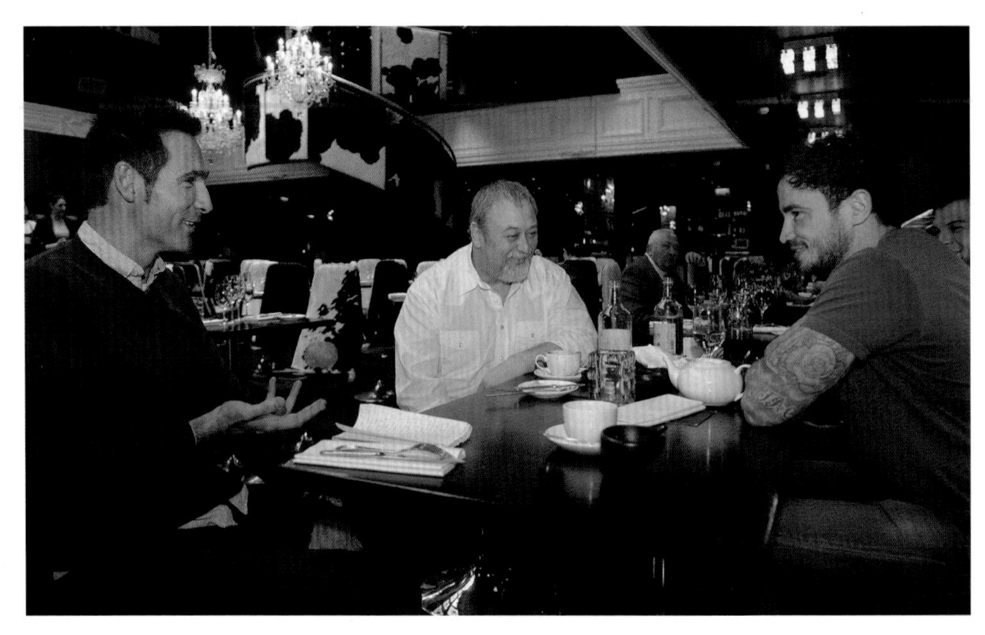

'Blackie' was like a father to me. I miss him dearly.

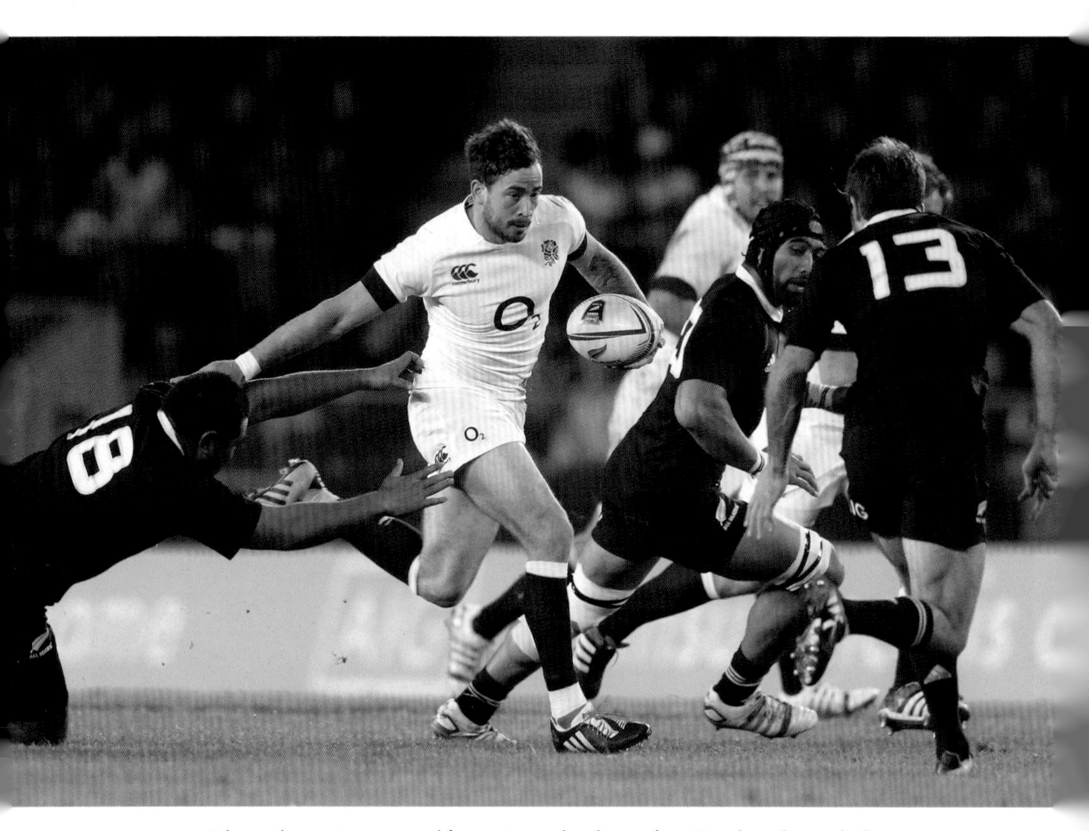

I loved testing myself against the best for England, and there are few better sides than New Zealand.

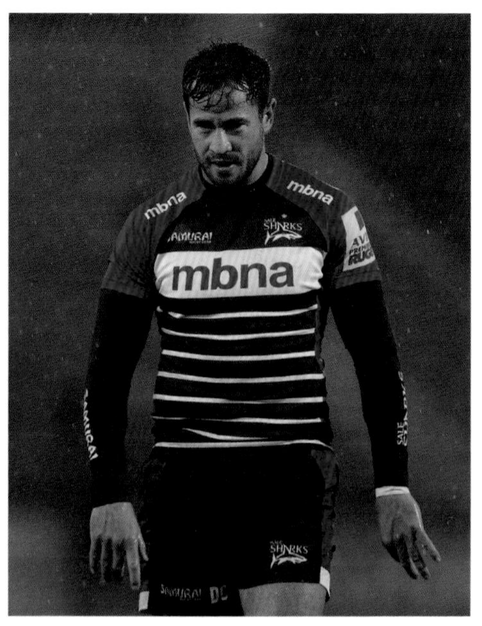

Playing for Sale Sharks against Newcastle Falcons on a rainy November day, 2015.

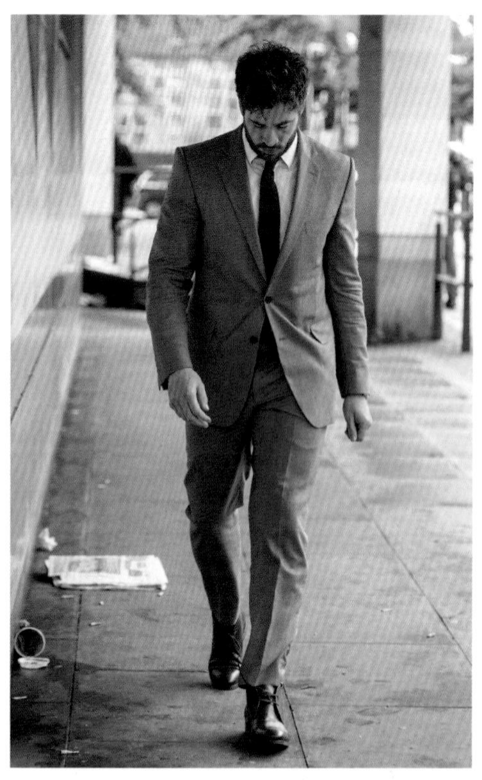

Leaving Westminster Magistrates' Court in June 2016.

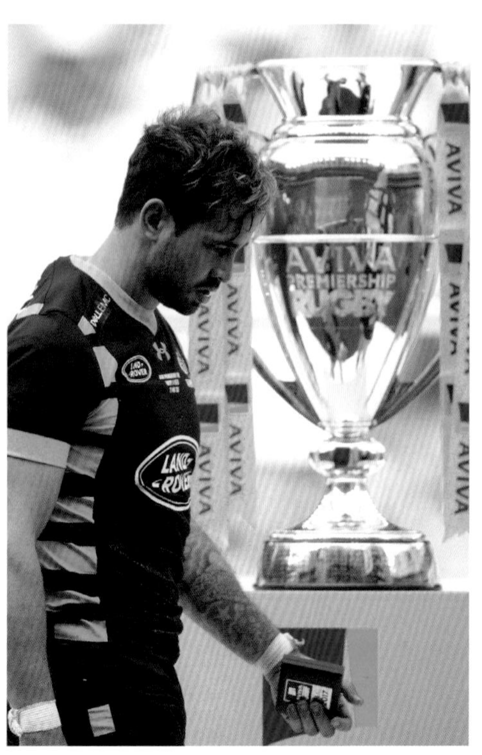

A close defeat by Exeter in the 2017 Premiership final really stung.

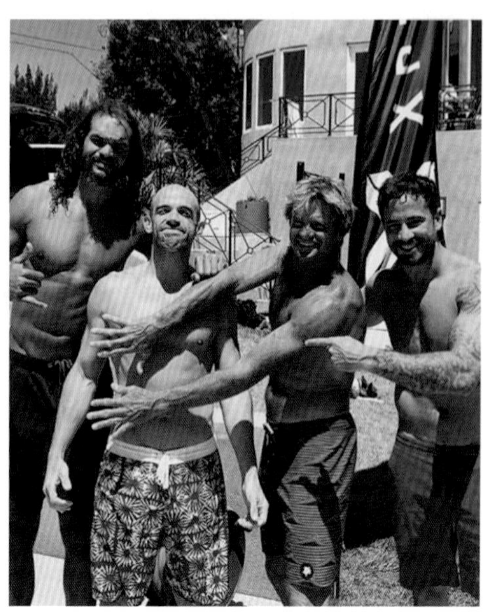

Hanging out with legends Joakim Noah, James Williams and Laird Hamilton in Malibu.

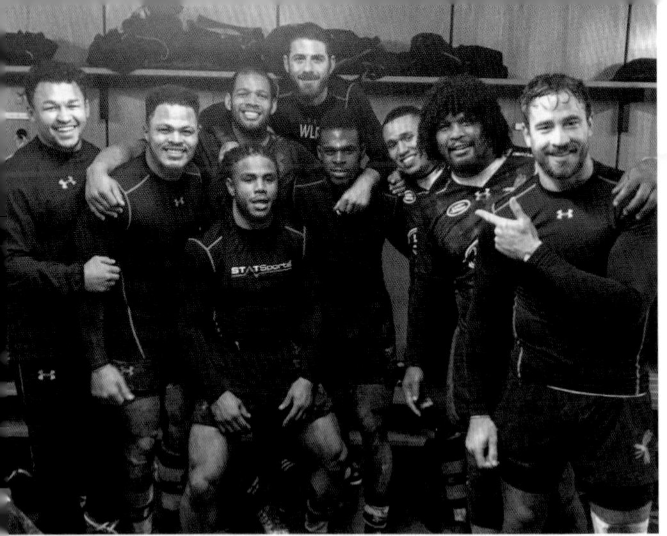

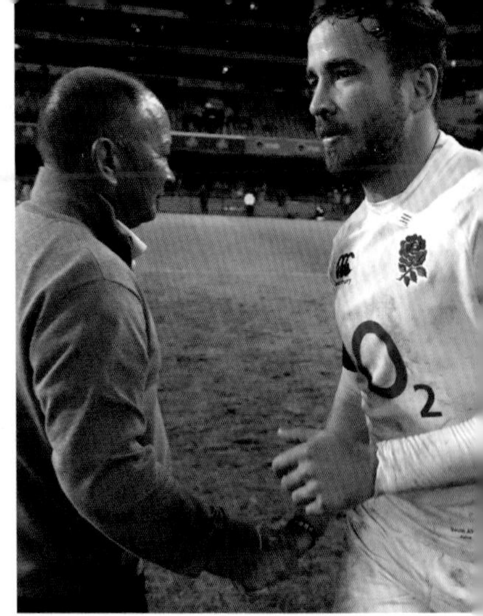

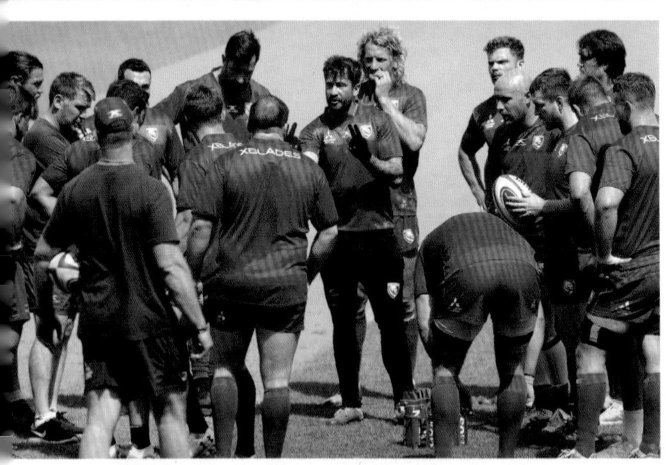

Top left: Creating memories with my 'Brothers' in the Wasps changing room, 2018.

Top right: We didn't see eye to eye, but I always gave my all for England, playing under Eddie Jones.

Left: Getting my message across to the boys at training with Gloucester in 2019.

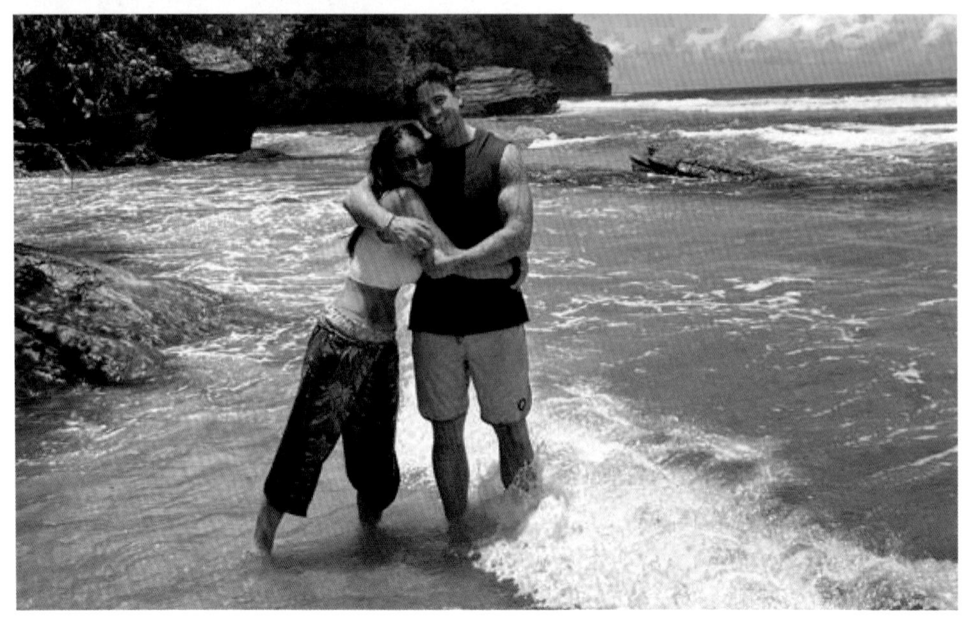

In Trinidad with my forever girl, Victoria Rose.

half, a new centre – but I'm left on the bench. When the final whistle goes, we're still 10 points down. And I'm thinking, *What was that about?*

As I'm walking down the tunnel, Andy Farrell gives me a pained smile, ruffles my hair and walks off looking dejected. I don't say a word. I'm still stunned they didn't put me on.

While I can't say for certain what's gone on, I have my theories. If I'd come on and done something special, Andy and Lanny would have been in an excruciating position. Even if we'd just come close to winning, people would have been saying, 'Why wasn't Cipriani introduced earlier? Surely he's got to start the next one? Surely he's got to play in the World Cup? Surely he's got the X-factor you need?'

As it is, Andy and Lanny won't have to answer those difficult questions. They can just put it down to a bad day at the office and carry on as before. Owen is our number one, George is our number two and Cipriani simply hasn't shown enough.

I get four minutes in the win over Scotland and come on late as a full-back in the crazy 55–35 win over France, which means we finish second in the table behind Ireland. But despite my frustrations, when I take to social media to say how much I've enjoyed it, I'm telling the truth.

I wish I'd been given more of a chance, but I still feel privileged and grateful. I love the professionalism of an international environment, waking up early, working on my skills, even the long meetings. After an England camp, I always return to my club with a new lease of life.

Probably because I've been doing the only thing I ever wanted, which is playing for my country.

Sale finish seventh in the Premiership, one place worse than last time. Outside the play-offs, but still good enough for a European spot.

That's quite an achievement, seeing as the club's owners have stopped putting as much money in, we've got fewer star players than a couple of years earlier and we're relying heavily on youngsters. On paper, we should have been scrapping for relegation.

Now I've been given the chance to run the show for England against the Barbarians. Happy days. I get the sense that England's coaches can't really be arsed, because it's not a proper Test match. But getting on with things without them works for me. Whenever that happens and I've got good players around me, I know what's going down.

I'm on it in training, making sure everyone knows exactly what he's doing and is feeling the same vibes as me. It's important we're not too loose and get things right, but it's not the normal highly-strung rugby union environment that makes players scared of expressing themselves – 'Don't do that! Do it like this! And if you can't get it right, don't do it at all!' – it's more a case of, 'It doesn't matter if you get it wrong, let's learn from it and go again.'

The Barbarians line-up is loaded with talent, including Australia's George Smith, who's got almost as many Test caps as our whole team put together, and All Black greats Brad Thorn, Sam Whitelock and Joe Rokocoko. But I score 31 points, including two tries, and we hammer them 73–12.

People will gloss over it – 'It's only the BaBas!' – but it's proof that if the vision and framework match, and each player understands his role in the team, while also being free to make their own decisions, the possibilities are endless.

After the game, me and some team-mates go for dinner on the King's Road, before I abandon my car and head onto a nightclub for drinks.

I'm buzzing about the game, and excited to be heading into the off-season, but it's nothing major, just a few cocktails, before rounding things off with an early morning breakfast. Then I'll drive straight home, pick up my bag and head to the airport, before catching a flight to LA.

As I'm rounding a corner at about 7 a.m., I stupidly check my phone, veer slightly, readjust too late, and a taxi coming in the other direction clips me. My car won't move. God knows what's happened to it, because when I get out to check the damage, there's barely a mark on it.

The taxi driver's screaming and shouting and I'm trying to get him to calm down, telling him we'll sort it out between us. I point out that all four of my wheels are in my lane, which means he must have swerved into me, not the other way around. But he pulls out his phone and calls the police.

The police can smell alcohol, so they put me in the back of their car and breathalyse me. It's been hours since my last drink, but I'm over the limit. At the station, they stick me in a cell and lock the door. *Oh, Danny*, I think, *what have you done now?* That's the thing about acting on impulse, it usually works great on a rugby field, but keeps getting me into strife off it.

I'm let out on bail, so I get a cab home, change my flight, head to the airport and cross my fingers. Even before I've taken off there's a report on the internet. One day I'm the toast of Twickenham, the next I'm very much not.

18

TRYING TO BE TRUE

I'm sitting in the sauna, it's hotter than the sun, and there are wise people everywhere I look. Writers, philosophers, scientists, athletes, actors, all high achievers, people with interesting perspectives they're only too happy to share.

The papers back in England assume I've come to California to party with celebs or had some sort of breakdown and become a hippy. Truth is, I've been doing this for a few years already, spending my summers in Malibu, hanging out with some of the most interesting people you could hope to meet. I used to spend my off-seasons getting out of my mind, now I spend them learning about my mind.

I stay with the big-wave surfer Laird Hamilton, his wife Gabby, who's half-Trinidadian like me, and their beautiful kids, plus whoever else happens to be in town. I was introduced to Laird and Gabby by my friend James Williams, who's heavily involved with Floyd Mayweather's business operations. The first time James asked me to join him, I had a terrible hangover and really couldn't be arsed. But I went and it changed my life.

This time Laird's been teaching me different types of breath work, which he learned from Dutch extreme athlete

Wim Hof, and I've also been doing some boxing with one of Manny Pacquiao's coaches. Laird is the most alpha male in the most extreme sport, yet is a great father to his girls and always willing to give his time and words of wisdom to anyone wanting to learn or in need. But the thing I love most is the conversation, which takes my mind to places it's never been. I've always been searching, felt there was more, and I feel extremely grateful to have met some exceptional characters with colourful life stories and a common zest for life.

Mostly, I sit and soak it all up. One day it's the writer Neil Strauss, a fascinating man who speaks wisely about parenting. Darin Olien is extremely detailed about nutrition and looks like Hercules. It blows my mind that he is vegan. Josh Brolin is a beautiful soul who has experienced the full spectrum of life, and I find comfort in talking with him. Orlando Bloom is a gentle character, a kindred spirit. Hutch Parker, who became a big brother to me, is always leading with his chest and looking out for me. And there's Sean Penn, who keeps popping out of the sauna for a cigarette, which Laird isn't a fan of. The record producer Rick Rubin is another fellow traveller, and when he speaks, you listen.

At a party one night, me and NBA player Blake Griffin chat for hours. Like me, Blake was a teenage prodigy, tipped for greatness. Also like me, his journey hasn't been as smooth as many people expected. But he's now a four-time NBA All-Star, and it's great having such an in-depth, vulnerable conversation with someone who's done and keeps doing such great things.

Blake explains that in the NBA, the relationship between coaches and players is usually less hierarchical, more open and honest. Everyone can speak, from the head coach down to the rookies, and everyone is listened to. I suspect that's why basketball has progressed so quickly and drastically, because the ideas of youngsters, who grew up in a different environment and view the world differently, are assimilated rather than discarded.

As a coach everyday life is a lot easier if it's your way or the highway. Some coaches will let youth have its say, but only pretend to listen. They don't want to hear new ideas in case they're good ideas, which they worry will force them to question old ideas they believed to be sacrosanct. And instead of a free-wheeling environment, they'll control meetings, like a schoolteacher.

Running meetings along the lines of a university tutorial, with everyone encouraged to chip in, can be hard going. But people will learn not to speak up for the sake of it, and only say something if it has some substance. And over time, those kinds of meetings will bear a bountiful supply of fruit.

In the NBA, it's all about being fully accepted for being yourself. To Blake, that's common sense. If a player is allowed to be himself, he'll be relaxed and limber, which is what you need to be if you want to excel at basketball. But in rugby union, coaches are hellbent on hammering players into a shape of their liking, and obsessed with the macho, yeoman bullshit. *Be aggressive! Get in their faces! Hit hard! Put your body on the line!* That sort of stuff just makes people tense, and it's severely limiting what rugby could be.

Making the situation worse is a media that loves picking apart people who are different, creating narratives around them and turning them into grotesque caricatures. These people are very mixed up, because there's an expectation for us to behave like wood off the field but water on it.

Spending time at Laird and Gabby's is like being plugged into an oracle and receiving an information download. But you know the craziest thing? It doesn't matter how intelligent someone is, they listen to what I have to say and seem genuinely interested.

People have preconceived ideas about these types of gatherings, that it's a load of blowhards spewing quasi-philosophy around a campfire. But that's not the case. I never feel intimidated, even when a guy who won a Nobel Prize for redefining the second, which sounds like something Dr Evil's dad would have done, is telling us how he did it. Somehow, he makes it relatable.

It's just a bunch of beautiful, humble souls who are open to the idea that there might be other ways. I feel their love and respect.

This is about as far away from Laird's place as it's possible to be. Miles and miles of running in the thin Colorado air, everyone in pieces, their bodies screaming. Mind-expanding it isn't. I feel like I'm back in the Dark Ages.

Whenever I return from LA and go back to rugby, it's like I'm at the bottom of the same hill I've been climbing for years. But this takes absurdity to whole new depths. Ridiculous amounts of running, constant fitness tests, a total waste of time. But I can't complain. Lanny's forgiven me, while others have been jettisoned for lapses in discipline, including Dylan Hartley for headbutting an opponent and Manu Tuilagi for assaulting some coppers. I've made it by the skin of my teeth, so I'm getting my head down and saying nothing.

It was a good idea to take the England team away, and the place we're staying, a ski resort called Vail, is great. We're in a lovely hotel and we can walk about unrecognised. It's the content of the trip that's letting us down.

After a running session, they'll ask us to play 15 v 15, and the quality is woeful because everyone is knackered. I don't think we've played any decent rugby since we arrived. The tone is set by Andy Farrell, which means everything is based on emotion. Andy's a big personality with a commanding presence, so no-one wants to confront him, including Lanny.

When Andy asks us to do something, everyone does it, no questions asked. And it's mostly to do with working harder and getting fitter – 'Fuckin' 'ell! We need more than this, boys!' – which is draining the life out of us.

I'll give you an example of the madness: they've started recording how long players spend on the floor and how quickly they get back on their feet. They've even created a list! Chris Robshaw is top, the best getter-upper in the squad. No wonder he's captain.

If you tell a group of athletes, 'This is what you need to do in order to be seen and picked', however mindless it is, that's all most of those athletes will think about. But I'm thinking, *Who gives a shit? Surely it's more important what they do when they're actually on their feet?*

Meanwhile, the coaches are wondering why our rugby is so poor.

I'm leading fitness tests, giving it my all in the gym, and doing everything to the letter of the law. But I'm doing it because I have to, not because it makes sense. Running hard and lifting heavier weights have their place, but they don't necessarily make you a better rugby player, they're just an easy way of providing stats and making it look like we're improving.

The coaches seem to think that if we can run more than other teams, we're fitter. But it doesn't work like that. Rugby isn't based on one-pace running, it's a repeat speed sport, so that's how you should train.

Compare our training to American football: all their training is tailored to individual players in specific positions, because different positions require different kinds of fitness. But they don't do that in rugby, maybe because too many rugby players are used to being told exactly what to do and scared of taking individual responsibility.

I've hit it off with Sam Burgess, who's been brought over from rugby league. Like me, Sam realises things aren't right. 'It's meetings about meetings,' he says. 'Why is everyone being treated like kids?' He's bang on, it feels like we're on a school trip rather than preparing for a World Cup.

Lanny's obviously read all the right books, and is a whizz with a whiteboard, but he's not big on *feel*. All this stuff about putting pride and passion back into the Red Rose – 'DO IT FOR ENGLAND AND ST GEORGE!' – sounds great to some people. But pride and passion in abstract things like symbols has got nothing to do with playing good rugby. It's performative, and means nothing when you step over that white line on match day.

If you pick 15 players for England, put them on a field in front of 80,000 fans, including their friends and family, and pay them 25 grand, of course there's going to be pride and passion on display, of course they're going to show willing. But it's a coach's job to channel that pride, passion and willing into a calm, enjoyable environment in which people can learn and grow together, so that when they're on the field, they feel united and confident enough to deliver the things you've been practising so hard in training.

If they're playing exciting rugby which the fans and media are lapping up, you don't even have to mention culture, passion and pride, all that stuff will happen naturally, because they'll desperately want to remain part of it. It's not difficult, but it does require emotional intelligence and trust in oneself. You have to really understand the intricacies of the game to set a team up like that. You have to really understand people, really have a *feel* for things.

There's been a lot of chat in the media about whether Sam should be here, seeing as he's only been in union for one season. Personally, I'm happy he's involved. He's got mad confidence in his own ability and is a great lad who gets on with everyone. What I find fascinating is how respected he is by Andy and Stuart, purely based on what he's achieved in league. When Sam talks in meetings, everyone falls silent, including those two.

The first chance we get, Sam and I, plus a few others, decide to escape the intensity and let our hair down. Going out is not strictly against the rules, but what we get up to is. We're at a strip club when we find out about a house party in Denver, so we jump on the back of some guy's pickup truck and head on over. Me and Sam are wrestling all the way there, and we can't stop laughing. It sounds dangerous, and it is, but it feels like a necessary release.

We've been at the party about 10 minutes when Sam starts feeling sick. Too much Jack Daniel's. But thank God for that, because we head back to the hotel and manage to slip into our rooms without being spotted.

Everyone knows there's a clique of players which helps run the team: Owen, George Ford, Chris Robshaw, Dan Cole, Ben Youngs, a couple of others. They're called 'the leadership group', but they're more like the mafia, always appearing to be scheming. Still, I get on fine with most of them. At least I think I do.

Sam's in a WhatsApp group with the mafia, until one day, he posts a picture on Instagram of me and him in a coffee shop. A few hours later, George screenshots the picture and messages it to Sam, before removing him from the group. Sam couldn't care less, but I think, *I'm not sure what I've done to offend them, but clearly I'm not as welcome as I thought I was.*

Will Greenwood, who won the World Cup with England, writes a column claiming my England team-mates don't like me. Sounds like it's probably true. I can only assume players are slagging me off in their mafia meetings and someone is leaking the contents of those conversations to the media, because nobody's said they've got an issue with me, just as nobody's ever said they've got an issue with me in an England environment.

It reminds me of when I was recovering from my terrible injury in 2008 and a mate said he'd lend me his Ferrari for a month as soon as I started running again. The day after my first running session with Kevin, this mate dropped the Ferrari off at my house. And a few weeks later, I drove it to an off-season England camp. Sacks, who's a big car guy, was almost drooling over it, and everyone else seemed cool. But fast forward three years and Lewis Moody is slagging me off about it in his memoir, claiming it was *an insight into what made Danny tick*. In other words, I'd got ideas above my station.

It feels pretty narrow-minded to judge a team-mate based on what car he drove to training one day. In football, nobody would ever suggest a player's car made any difference to how committed they were. Last time I checked, Cristiano Ronaldo was driving around in a £1 million Bugatti, and I'm not sure there's a more committed sportsman in the world.

The coaches seem to think that because everyone's returned from Colorado in bits, the camp has gone well. But I can't say many of the players are doing cartwheels.

Rugby players moan about everything, but that's not necessarily a good thing. Being a professional rugby player should be the best time of our lives. We should be having inspiring conversations, doing innovative things in training, going to bed every night thinking, *Wow, I learned so much today*. Instead, everyone's flat-out exhausted, and while they're too afraid to say anything to the coaches, I suspect a lot of them are wondering if we're heading in the right direction, if things should be done differently, if we're being set up to fail.

We've reconvened at Pennyhill Park and Andy's setting up drills so there'll be as few line breaks as possible, because he wants our defence to rule.

When a line break does happen, I'm often involved, usually creating a hole for someone else. But I'm struggling to understand why they've decided to tighten things up. We played some expansive rugby towards the end of the Six Nations, but it's suddenly turned safe and heavily stats-based. Plus, you've got Lanny doing his patriotic thing, and Andy, who's heavily involved in defence and attack, overloading every meeting with emotion, which is extra baggage.

I think back to my conversation with Blake Griffin and how things are done in the NBA. Basketball isn't a collision sport like rugby, but it's incredibly physically demanding, what with the amount of games they play and all that jumping, landing and swivelling. However, you can't be a top NBA player on physical attributes alone, you have to have sublime ball-playing skills as well.

For those skills to flow, you have to be loose and relaxed. And to be loose and relaxed, and therefore better at making decisions, you have to enjoy what you're doing, understand that it's just a game, not life or death. But this England camp feels like we're about to be invaded by a foreign army.

Lanny tells the press I need to shine in the warm-up games to have any chance of being in the final squad, but I only get half an hour in the first one against France at Twickenham. I play full-back and only touch the ball once.

Before the return game in Paris, I speak to my modelling agent Vanessa, who's quite spiritual. She tells me about ancestors and how they live on in your body, through their DNA. 'Whenever you think you're alone', she says, 'you're not, because your ancestors are with you.' We went quite deep, and I came away from that chat with a sense of belonging I hadn't experienced often.

For a long time, I'd looked outside for validation – from Mum and Dad in particular – and not got it. Blackie and the guys in Malibu taught me that I can find validation internally, and now Vanessa had taught me that even when you feel empty as hell, you're brimming with the power of your forebears.

In Paris, I'm still on the bench halfway through the second half, and we're getting hammered. Often when the camera cuts to the bench, the replacements will be chatting and laughing. But Blackie's taught me to stay mentally engaged, so that I'm in the game, thinking about what I would have done in every scenario. And if I am introduced, I'll be up to speed immediately.

When they finally decide to give me a run after 63 minutes, the camera shows me looking at the coaches, and it's not difficult to see what's going through my mind: *Don't you think I can do anything in 17 minutes? Fuck you ...* I just feel so good, so focused, so locked into the moment.

I'm on at full-back, but still manage to catch the eye. The tempo increases, we've suddenly got some zip, and I score our first try with eight minutes remaining. A bit of footwork, slowing down to sow doubt in the defender's mind, then speeding up and powering over the line. Another late try makes the scoreline look respectable, 25–20 to France, but apart from those final 17 minutes, it's been a dismal performance.

I'm voted man of the match and most people seem to think I've done enough to secure my place in the final World Cup squad. Maybe as a utility player, someone who can cover a few positions, but I'd take it. But as I'm leaving the press room after my man-of-the-match interview, I hear Lanny being asked about my performance. 'Danny was good,' he says, 'but everyone else who came on was good as well.' That's when I knew they'd already made their minds up.

Over the next few days, the papers are full of articles calling for my inclusion. The *Sun* goes with 'PICK CIPS – Danny's got the X-factor.' The *Express* calls me 'the player England desperately need'. The *Independent* says, 'Cipriani looked a world-beater when compared to the majority of his countrymen.' The *Times* says, 'To ignore Cipriani is to ignore the evidence of the two games against France.' Clive Woodward, Will Greenwood, Lawrence Dallaglio and Dean Ryan all back me. But it's Eddie Butler in the *Guardian* who seems the most perceptive: 'Did England ever want Cipriani to be an answer?' he says.

Lanny breaks the bad news to me the following Tuesday. He's only picked two fly-halves, Owen and George, and he's gone with Mike Brown and Alex Goode at full-back.

I say to him, 'You copped out, mate. You never even played me at 10. But I did all I could and I respect your decision.' And that was the end of it. Other players who get bombed out have meetings that last half an hour.

I've just been told I'm not in the World Cup squad and now I'm pushing a heavy sled around the field. It's mindless, as dumb as it gets, but I'm mucking in because I don't want my team-mates to suffer more than they need to.

Suddenly, our attack coach Mike Catt screams, 'For fuck's sake, Danny, put your back into it!' I don't say anything, but I give him a puzzled look and think, *What the fuck is his problem?*

Catt's had beef with me for years. He's slagged me off in the papers, called me a liability, and he once whacked me around the head when I was playing for Wasps and he was playing for London Irish. When the final whistle went, I refused to shake his hand, and his team-mates accused me of being a dickhead. But as far as I was concerned, it was all water under the bridge.

I get back to pushing this sled, a bit of anger in me now, and a couple of minutes later, Catt comes at me again: 'Fucking hell, Danny, is that the best you can do?' I stop what I'm doing, give him my best *Don't you fucking speak to me like that* stare and get back to pushing, but my heart's not in it now.

I'm thinking, *They've just told me I'm not playing in the World Cup and now this wanker's taking the piss out of me*. Then it happens again – 'Fucking shit, Danny, work harder!' – and this time I've had more than enough.

I walk straight towards him, get in his face and say, 'Have you got something to say to me, Mike Catt?' He starts stuttering, before screaming in my face, spittle flying everywhere, 'As long as I'm involved, you'll never play for England again!'

There's a short, but very pregnant, pause. Then I say, 'You've just shown your true colours,' before walking off. Everyone's stopped what they're doing and there's a very uncomfortable hush. As I'm walking off, Lanny's all in a tizz: 'What's going on? Why did he say that?' I say to him, 'Go and ask him.'

Some of my team-mates aren't happy and tell Catt he's been out of order. Joe Marler and Dan Cole, who were pushing the same sled as me, say I was putting my fair share in. Chris Robshaw asks me if I'm okay. They're very sensitive to the situation, understand how I must have been feeling about being dropped, even before Catt got stuck into me. It looked blatantly unjust, like straight-up bullying. And people tend not to like injustice or bullies.

I'm trying to be true to myself and I've got people like Mike Catt trying to paint me as some sort of trouble-maker. Fuck that. I don't care who you are, an England coach or Lord God Almighty, you don't speak to anyone like that.

But when the story is leaked, I get the blame. It doesn't matter that I tell the press it was just one of those things, and that me and Mike Catt have a good working relationship, because I don't want to disrupt England's World Cup preparations. I have to be the problem, because the truth doesn't fit the narrative they've been spinning for the best part of a decade.

19

WHAT DID I JUST SEE?

Getting man of the match at Twickenham and done for drink driving on the way home certainly didn't help my cause. But I'm not sure it made much difference in the grand scheme of things. The fact I trained mostly at full-back, and barely got a sniff in the warm-up games, tells me everything I need to know.

If they'd given me 40 minutes or more at fly-half and I'd played the house down, that would have put them in a bit of a bind. They'd have been under intense pressure from the media, with journalists and ex-players saying I must be picked, and Andy and Lanny would have had to rethink their four-year plan at the last minute.

When Andy is asked about my 17-minute man-of-the-match display against France, he says they couldn't pick a player based on one small piece of evidence and that selection has to be based on facts, not perception, and has to be right for the group.

I get that he has to say something, because journalists keep asking about me, but how does his explanation make sense? It's a fact that I won man of the match, not a perception. He calls it a perception because my performance didn't align with his plans. And publicly questioning my character and integrity is an archaic, bully-boy mentality.

Instead of saying I'm not right for the group, why not just say they felt other players fitted better with what they were trying to do on the field? Besides, I behaved impeccably in camp.

Rugby is supposed to be a professional sport, but there's nothing professional about what's happened. The coaches took a group of lads who were beginning to gel and play some eye-catching rugby and ground the life out of them. And while Andy is a very good technical coach, one of the best I've had, he's too emotionally invested, which is clouding his judgement.

Sam Burgess is a great lad and a brilliant rugby player, but how can selection be based on facts, rather than perception, when he's only started a handful of games at centre for Bath and was switched to back-row at the end of the season? I'm not saying Sam shouldn't be in the squad, but he's being judged by different standards to me. It's almost impossible not to take things personally.

I write a magnanimous Instagram post, wishing the boys good luck and telling the country to get behind them, and that's truly how I feel. But in private, I can't help thinking, *Is this really the sport for me?*

But I have to bury the anger, bitterness and resentment, because that's the only way to move forward. A few days after the England squad announcement, I meet with

Blackie and we put together a plan, focusing on getting even better the following season and back into the England team.

Diversity and inclusion aren't just about how people look and sound, it's about how people think. At least it should be. Doing what's best means having frank, honest conversations with people who see the world differently and make you feel uncomfortable, because confrontation and friction often lead to growth. On the other hand, actively avoiding confrontation and friction, because it looks like the right thing to do, often leads to stagnation.

It takes courage to leave your comfort zone, try things that people are going to be suspicious of, rip up old traditions that people hold dear. But only by doing that are you going to find out who you are and what you can do, as well as produce players who think and do things differently on the field.

I'm certainly not the only player who has been let down by the English way of doing things. In fact, there are always about five players who should be getting a look in but aren't, and about five players in the squad who should be nowhere near it. And that goes for club rugby as well as the England set-up.

Sport is an expression of art, but unlike in art, greatness in sport is quantifiable. A player is either doing great things for his club or he isn't. But England coaches are too much like art critics, in that they pick based on personal preference, on how someone's work fits into their view of the world.

I'm a fly-half, eager to learn and lead, so I need and want to sit at the front of meetings and contribute. But most blokes who sit at the front of meetings and contribute end up in leadership groups, which usually means parroting the coaches' message, rather than offering alternative points of view.

On the flip side, those blokes who sit silently at the back, maybe because they're more introverted, might have something far more interesting to say than those in the leadership group. But the coaches are never going to ask them for their opinion, and they're less likely to get picked for the team. There's also the primeval fear of being ostracised from the group, which in tribal times would mean death.

When Lanny banned us from wearing headphones while we were walking into Twickenham, because he wanted us to soak up the atmosphere and connect with the fans – which is a nice sentiment – someone in the leadership group should have said, 'You know what, Stuart, I don't agree.'

A player should be able to do whatever makes him most comfortable and ready for the game to come. If he wants to cartwheel off the bus and go round high-fiving fans, let him do it. If he wants to stare at the ground and wear headphones, because he's listening to relaxing music or voice notes, or simply wants to block out any distractions, let him do that as well. Players can't be worrying about being seen to do the right thing, and they can't be worrying about what the fans think, because if they're doing that, they're not really being themselves. Before the game has even kicked off, you're acting.

As it was, no-one said anything, because they saw their job as reinforcing Lanny's message. But I guarantee you some of them were thinking, *Why do the coaches feel the need to dictate to us? How can they possibly know what's best for individuals?* This isn't management, this is control and the fear of what might happen if anyone strays from your strictures.

Everyone's going on about Sam being picked ahead of Northampton's Luther Burrell, who was an ever-present in England's last two Six Nations campaigns, but I reckon Kyle Eastmond had an even better claim.

Kyle played for Bath in the Premiership final, while Sam was in the back-row. He's a special player, doing things at 12 that no-one else in England is doing – putting people into space and using his electric change of speed to play around people, rather than always trying to blast through the middle. If England had that option at 12, as well as 10, they could split the field and be so dangerous in attack. Instead, they're fixated on physical dominance.

It probably hasn't helped Kyle that he's an outspoken lad from Oldham. If he feels he's being treated badly, he can get angry, shout and spew. Most coaches would say he's hard to manage, but he's a really good fella, smart, with a big heart. If England's coaches tried to understand him better, you'd see a player doing some crazy things on the field.

Saracens wing Chris Ashton is a great finisher, and maybe should have been selected, but I'm more shocked that Christian Wade wasn't even in the conversation, because he can't stop scoring tries, and there's no other winger that can do what Wadey does. Someone like Jonny May will do sensational things three or four times a season, but Wadey does sensational things two or three times a game, stuff that makes you think, *What did I just see?*

People are always talking about his apparent weaknesses, rather than his strengths. They say he's too small, but his tackling is fine. They say he can't defend box kicks, but that's simply not true. But any coach worth his salt wouldn't select based on fear, they would select on what could be.

The question the England coaches should be asking is, 'Is any English winger better than Wadey at beating defenders?' To which the answer is no. With ball in hand, he can have almost every winger in the world for breakfast, lunch and dinner, and all the other parts of the game are easily coachable.

I'll tell you a story about Wadey that might go some way to explaining things. When he was on tour with the Lions in 2013, they panned to him in the crowd during a game and he started combing his hair with his Afro comb. He wasn't even in the match squad, but the next time he was in the England set-up, Lanny had a go at him for messing about.

Wadey couldn't believe it – 'What's that got to do with anything?' – but that's English rugby for you. It doesn't want players to reveal their true personalities, even if by doing so they can produce magic.

I can't help thinking of the basketball player Steph Curry and the warm-ups he does before games. He laughs and jokes, does insane things with the ball, including kicking it through the hoop. If a rugby player was seen warming up like that, they'd get a bollocking. 'Stop taking the piss, start taking the game seriously, you're far too loose.' But it certainly works for Steph.

If Lanny wanted to put passion back into the England jersey and make the country proud, it didn't look much like it.

What went wrong? A lot of things. For more than three years, the coaches tried to build a decision-making game-plan. But after the 2015 Six Nations, in which England scored 18 tries, they switched to a more physical, direct approach, thinking they could suddenly become South Africa.

In the losses to Wales and Australia, you could tell that players weren't playing instinctively, they were second-guessing themselves. The coaches changing their philosophy so late in the day bred uncertainty throughout the squad. Far from looking like the fittest team in the tournament, they were off the pace and sluggish, probably because of the neanderthal training in the build-up and the unnecessary emotional pressure piled on by the coaches.

But the seeds of England's sorry early exit were sown years ago. If you stand still in sport, because you want to remain safe in your comfort zone, you're in serious trouble. Football is always evolving because the best coaches are terrified of being caught up by the rest of the field and swamped. But those in charge of English rugby seemed to want to hold onto the past for as long as possible – and now it's fallen and smashed into a thousand pieces.

BRIAN ASHTON

When I started England's National Academy, it was meant to be a group of 16 to 19-year-olds who might go on to play for the senior team. But I was also looking for players who brought something different, who didn't adhere to the traditional, conservative English way of playing rugby.

I first saw Danny playing for England Under-15s against Italy, and he immediately sparked my interest. And when I invited him to join the Academy, when he was still only 15, boy did he show he was different.

Despite being the youngest, he was very confident, and courageous when it came to trying new things. Some of the older guys had already experienced professional rugby, so were used to the idea that youngsters sat at the back and kept quiet. But Danny sat at the front and never shut up.

That didn't go down well with all of his team-mates, but I loved it. I didn't want players to just sit and listen, I wanted them to have opinions and challenge the status quo. Because only when people challenge the status quo do you make progress.

I'd coached a lot of talented players down the years, but not many as talented as Danny. Part of the reason he thought differently was probably because of his unconventional upbringing. But what really set him apart, and made him try all sorts of crazy things, was the fact he was a fantastic all-round games player – he probably could have played football or cricket professionally – which made him multi-dimensional and 'game intelligent'.

One of my mottos is 'practise in the notion of impossibility'. That means if a player comes up with an idea that seems unworkable, we practise it anyway. It might not work, but something might come of it that does. That's collaborative coaching – coaches and players working out things together, instead of coaches simply telling players how to play.

But the kind of intelligence Danny had, which meant he liked experimenting and understood how to change games mid-flow, is unusual nowadays, because talented kids are too often encouraged to concentrate on one sport from an early age, and only do what the coach tells them.

I got plenty of stick when I dropped Danny for the game against Scotland, when he was photographed leaving a nightclub. He told me he hadn't been drinking, and I believed him. But I didn't think it was acceptable, and I thought I did the right thing. He was pissed off, but when I told him he was starting against Ireland the following weekend, I meant what I said.

An inexperienced player asking to run a session a few days before an international is pretty unusual, but I'd known Danny for five or six years by then, so it wasn't as outrageous as it might sound. When I asked if he was sure, he said to me, 'Do you want me to lead the team on Saturday?'

I cleared it with the captain Phil Vickery, who was Danny's team-mate at Wasps, and we ran Wednesday's attack session together. But Danny had as much input as I did, and when he had something to say, I stood back.

A coach should be a facilitator, a consigliere, and players should be given licence to read and interpret situations as they see fit, because they're the ones who play the games. But it wasn't a case of Danny telling his team-mates what to do, it was more a conversation about how he wanted to play.

Danny's approach was observational and emotional, in that he wanted the team to play what they saw and how they felt, within a framework. And on the Saturday, Danny was unbelievable. He ripped Ireland apart.

When Danny swore in his post-match interview, I thought it was quite amusing, but the guys from the RFU were up in arms. I reminded them that he was a young lad who'd just been named man of the match on his starting debut for England. But Danny had replaced a god of English rugby in Jonny Wilkinson, and I imagine people from the RFU and in the media were thinking, *Is this the sort of person we want representing our country?*

Still, if you'd told me after that Ireland game that Danny would only win another 15 England caps, I'd have thought you were mad. Yes, he was forthright, honest and challenging. But I always found him challenging in a positive way. Why would you want a guy like Danny, who's got such a wide-ranging skillset and such a great imagination, to keep his ideas to himself? You don't move forward if you don't have positive disruptors in your group.

I sometimes watch England and think, *Is this really how they want to play the game? Is this really their authentic selves we're seeing?* But I never had that feeling watching Danny. One thing you could guarantee with Danny was that every time he played a game of rugby, that was really him.

Danny was doing remarkable things for various club sides for over a decade. And he wasn't flash, like some people thought he was, he was just consistently different. But English rugby doesn't really like difference, and too many coaches are fearful of the consequences of change. Instead of being excited about what might be, they worry about what might go wrong.

Had Danny been born in New Zealand, he'd have played a lot of games for the All Blacks. I think he'd have fitted in quite nicely. As it is, I fear Danny will be remembered as a great player who was wasted by the English game, because he didn't conform to what an English player was expected to be.

20

AT LEAST I'M TRYING

I thought I'd never make it past 27, like those rock stars and actors I'd read about who didn't feel enough, were harshly judged, or just felt like they didn't fit in. Not that I'm directly comparing myself to Jim Morrison, Kurt Cobain, Amy Winehouse or anyone else who left this world too soon, but I thought I'd stagger off in the wrong direction at some point, get hopelessly lost and topple off a cliff.

But every time I lose my bearings, someone appears out of the gloom, places a hand on my shoulder and leads me back to the right path. Shaun, Kevin, Margot, Luke and Mel in Melbourne, Laird in LA, Blackie of course.

Mum and Dad? Not so much. It feels like people are asking for cash and not much else, and I can't have honest conversations with Mum. No wonder my interactions with women are so shady, that I'm only interested in snatching what I want before running a mile.

But one evening in Malibu, I'm sat around a friend's dinner table, chatting about life, and my mind wanders back to the time my dad left. I'd never been able to speak about that moment without feeling exactly how I did at the time, as if part of my heart was being torn out, which is why I tried to avoid the subject. But on this occasion, for the first time, I didn't feel like that.

I saw things from a different perspective and realised that Dad leaving was him teaching me to be my own man. England wasn't for him, so he went home to Tobago, for the sake of his sanity and happiness. I wasn't suddenly giving him a pass – he had, after all, left his son behind – but reassessing and reshaping the past relieved the pain and lightened the intensity.

Opening myself up to multiple perspectives, rather than fixating on myself as the victim, meant I felt able to move on. It was as if I'd untangled myself from the past and was suddenly able to see clearly in the present.

England's new head coach Eddie Jones calls me in for a meeting. I'd been hoping for someone foreign, with a non-English mindset, so I'm quite excited. Plus, Eddie must rate me, because he tried to sign me when I was at Wasps and he was at Saracens.

No sooner have we shaken hands than he pulls out his laptop and sparks up footage of my 17-minute, man-of-the-match display against France. I think he's going to start waxing lyrical – *Play like this, mate, and you're my starting 10.* Instead, he says, in that whiny Aussie accent of his, 'Mate, you've got to be doing it like this instead. See what you've done there, mate? That's not going to work ...' I can't believe what I'm hearing. And I come out of the meeting thinking, *Jesus, I've got another fight on my hands ...*

The following month, Eddie announces his first squad for the 2016 Six Nations. Ten lads who played in the World Cup are dropped and seven uncapped players are called up. I'm not. When Eddie is asked why, he says I'm not good enough and need to work on various areas of my game. He doesn't even know me, yet it seems like his mind is already made up.

For years, I've been training to trust myself fully on a rugby field, and now I'm training to trust myself fully in the wider world. As well as working my body, I'm working my mind. I'm meditating, watching a lot of spiritual stuff on the internet and reading books by great thinkers. I've been reading since I was in my mid-20s, but only recently have I started feeling the words, working out what they really mean and how they might apply to my life.

I read about neuroscience and the possible origins of the universe. There's a Mexican guy I love called Don Miguel Ruiz, who uses ancient teachings to help people achieve spiritual enlightenment. It's not just what he says that I love about him, it's also how he says it. His books are simple, with no long words and difficult sentences. He's not trying to show off how clever he is, he just wants as many people as possible to understand themselves.

Before hanging out with my friends in Malibu, and reading Ruiz and others like him, I thought you had to be super-smart to learn from people like that. And when I say super-smart, I mean good A-levels and a university degree.

But now I realise that intelligence isn't about how much you can remember from books, it's deeper than that. It's wanting to grow, figure yourself out, better understand your mind and how it works. It's having the courage to face and forgive yourself and be accountable for your actions.

I'm acutely aware that my journey's not going to be easy, because while I'm growing as a person, I'm stuck in a sport that doesn't seem to want me to. Sometimes, I feel like one of those plants you see in jars, whose flowers are unable to open to their full extent.

I'm still popping Tramadol and sleeping with an awful lot of women. And I still haven't reached a point where I find peace just sitting and thinking. But I'm more aware that for real change to happen, it has to come from within.

Sale almost go unbeaten at home in the 2015–16 season. It's another top six finish and the undoubted highlight is playing with my old schoolmate Neville Edwards.

I'd watched Nev play for Rosslyn Park the previous summer and couldn't get my head around how so many clubs had passed on him – he had incredible footwork and such a good work ethic. So I said to him, 'Mate, with a bit of a steer on defensive positioning, you could play in the Premiership and thrive.' I arranged for him to have a trial with Sale, Dimes liked the look of him, and he's ended up being our top try-scorer this season.

Nev's dream was to play in the Premiership and now he's doing it, which has been great to see. But I also think about how much talent falls through the cracks, because too many people in rugby have the same erroneous idea of what a rugby player should look like.

I originally thought I'd give Sale another year, because Dimes was treating me well and I was enjoying my rugby. But my ambition is driving me, and if I want to play for England, I need to be playing for a club with a more dominant pack.

I'm about to sign for Harlequins when my agent tells me Wasps are interested. It's my boyhood club, there's an emotional attachment and they're building an exciting team. And when we meet head coach Dai Young in a hotel in Ealing, he tells me he needs me to run his attack, that I'm the perfect man to lead all these exciting players he's bringing in. So that's that, decision made, I tell my agent we're going to Wasps instead.

Dimes is sad to lose me but accepts my decision, at least in private. In public, he tells the media I've made a bad decision and he'll easily replace me. Rewind a couple of years and he's telling the media I'd be playing for England if I was at a bigger club, so he knows what's what.

A week after my move is announced, I score a late winner against title-chasing Leicester. 'It was a brilliant try, to be fair,' says Dimes, through gritted teeth.

Eddie's picked me for a three-day training camp at Pennyhill Park. We're all out for dinner on day one, I'm sitting at the end of the table and Eddie comes and sits next to me. The first words out of his mouth are, 'Mate, doesn't Kirsty Gallacher live around here? Haven't you shagged her? What's she like?'

I've just split up with Kirsty, after a short relationship, and it's not something I want to talk to my head coach about, or anyone else for that matter. Eddie keeps pecking, like a horny teenager, and in the end I tell him straight, 'Eddie, I don't want to talk about this, it's making me uncomfortable.'

Surprise, surprise, I'm not in the squad for the summer international against Wales. He's picked a part-time 10 ahead of me. I can't help thinking Eddie only picked me for that training camp as a joke.

I also miss out on the tour to Australia and end up in South Africa with the Saxons instead. Chris Ashton's turned the Saxons tour down, because he's upset at not being picked for the first team, but I'm well up for it, happy to take whatever route necessary to get back into England's first team.

All the talk about me being a bad tourist is nothing but a whispering campaign. I'm with a great group of lads, some of whom should be in Australia, including our two wingers. Wadey should have had 30 or 40 caps for England by now, while Semesa Rokoduguni won one cap against the All Blacks, played fine and hasn't been picked since. Those two games against South Africa A aren't easy, but we win both and everyone comes home happy.

I'm not back long when I get whacked with an 18-month ban and an eight grand fine for drink-driving. Next day, there's a made-up story about me dating a celebrity. The day after that, there's another one. When England's football team are knocked out of the European Championships by Iceland, it's almost a relief, because the media's guns are all trained on Roy Hodgson and his players instead.

Wasps' back-line for the 2016–17 season is full of deadly weapons and I can't wait to be a part of it. They already had Wadey, Elliot Daly and Dan Robson, all England internationals, but they've added Kyle Eastmond, my old mate Kurtley Beale and South Africa's Willie le Roux. On paper, it's terrifying.

Pre-season goes well, at least I think it has, until Dai sticks me on the bench for the final warm-up game against Bristol, with Jimmy Gopperth starting at 10. I ask Dai why I'm not starting, and he says, 'Jimmy's been training better than you.' I laugh and reply, 'That's not possible.'

It sounds arrogant, I know, but I've been training with Jimmy for a month and it's obvious his skillset is more suited to 12. Jimmy's a very good player, a reliable kicker, a strong runner, solid in defence, but he can't do what I do at fly-half, just as I can't do what he does at 12. Also, why would Dai beg me to sign and run the attack, and then when I've tried to do just that in training, put someone in ahead of me? I can only conclude that when he said he wanted me to run the attack, he meant he wanted me to run *his* attack.

It's half-time against Bristol and we're losing 9–0. Dai must be thinking, *Jesus, I've assembled one of the most expensive teams in the league and we're being made to look like mugs by a team that's just been promoted.* He puts me on with 20 minutes to go, we win the game, and afterwards Dai says, 'I'm gonna start you at 10 for the next one.'

With me at 10 and Jimmy at 12, we win our first five league games of the season, bumping off Exeter, Leicester, Bristol, Northampton and Harlequins, and scoring 26 tries in the process. Our back-line is even more terrifying in real life than it was on paper. I'm not thrilled that Jimmy's retained kicking duties, because I think I have to do everything to be considered for England. But Dai was already making me feel like he was doing me a favour by playing me at all, and Jimmy's keen, so I feel like it's best not to say anything.

Dai might not want me to run attack in training, but he doesn't really have a choice. Our backs coach Lee Blackett is pretty green, but he wears his heart on his sleeve and genuinely cares, which is rare. He also has an extremely experienced back line, so rather than imposing his ideas he offers some great insight and is also willing to listen even if his hands are sometimes tied from above.

It's not a case of the backs just chucking the ball around and hoping for the best. We have a framework, which consists of making sure the forwards are in the right place when we want to attack, with the front five and number eight in the middle of the field and back-rows on the edge. We always make sure the short side is loaded, and switch quickly to the open side if the short side is well defended. There are a lot of moving parts, but it's all clicking.

When we beat Bath on Christmas Eve, we've only lost two games out of 11. Wadey scores a brilliant hat-trick that day, and his second try is out of this world. By the time he's touched the ball down, there are Bath defenders on their backsides all over the field. To celebrate, we do a little dance.

At Tuesday's team meeting, Dai says, 'What was that on Saturday? An audition for *Britain's Got Talent*? I don't want to see anyone celebrating like that again.'

Poor Wadey, he's really upset. He asks for a meeting with Dai and tells him he feels belittled. Dai says that if he lets us get away with it, everyone will follow suit. Who cares?! Can you imagine Pep Guardiola telling Sergio Aguero not to celebrate? Or Raheem Sterling? They'd look at him like he'd lost his mind. Anyone who knows Wadey properly will say he's a lad with a big heart who likes to express himself. He wasn't doing a little dance because he wanted to rub the other team's noses in it, he was just having fun.

Not allowing players to react naturally to what should be a joyous moment is madness, because you're effectively telling them not to be themselves. And if a player can't be himself, he can't fulfil his potential. That's English rugby in a nutshell – needing to look a certain way, be seen to do things *properly*, even if doing things properly is holding you back.

Most people in rugby seem to be uncomfortable with displays of emotion, presumably because they associate emotion with weakness and femininity. The media are just as bad as the coaches, getting all sniffy any time a player gets carried away. But how can you condemn emotion, when it's emotion that makes someone human?

That condemnation reveals a lack of compassion and acceptance.

Wadey stops celebrating after that. Every time he scores, he just trots back to the halfway line. I think, *You've torn that kid's heart out.*

After leaving me out of his squad for the autumn internationals, Eddie says I'm only happy being *number one, the main man*, insinuating I'd be disruptive if I wasn't in the starting XV. Owen's injured, so his Saracens understudy Alex Lozowski, who left Wasps after I signed, is picked ahead of me.

Eddie has had two conversations with me, the first when he pulled apart my man-of-the-match display against France, the second when he wanted to know who I'd been shagging.

If he really got to know me, he'd realise I'd happily sit on the bench for England. If he wanted to understand what kind of team man I was, he'd speak to my Saxons coaches, Ali Hepher of Exeter and Alan Dickens of Northampton, who I got on great with in South Africa.

I can only conclude that Eddie doesn't want to understand, that's it's more convenient and easier for him to judge me on my past. Like Lanny and Andy before him, he knows that if I come off the bench and change the face of a game, there'll be a clamour for me to start the next one, including lots of awkward questions and conversations with the media that he'd rather not face.

Eddie is obviously irritated whenever a journalist mentions my name, but he never gives them a proper explanation as to why he's overlooked me. It always boils down to, 'My opinion is my opinion, and because it's my opinion, it's the right opinion. As for you lot, you don't know what you're talking about.'

I get the sense I make Eddie feel uncomfortable, even when I'm not there and people are just talking about me. Meanwhile, the guys he gets on best with tend to do exactly as they're told and keep quiet.

21

I AM WHAT I AM

I'm having the time of my life with Wasps. I'm enjoying living in Leamington Spa, just down the road from our ground in Coventry, where there's not much going on or trouble to get into, and I spend most days with a talented group of players who I get on great with.

The changing room is full of what we call 'the brothers' – me, Wadey, Kurtley, Kyle Eastmond, Nathan Hughes, Ashley Johnson, Juan de Jongh, Gaby Lovobalavu, Nizaam Carr and our honorary member Willie le Roux – and having that many black and brown faces around makes me feel more comfortable.

It's unusual, going through life as a mixed-race person who almost everyone assumes is white. When I was at school, kids would make racist jokes, not knowing my dad was from Trinidad, and I'd have to tell them not to say that kind of stuff around me. I was always into hip-hop, R&B, reggae, anything Dad listened to, and people would think I wanted to be black. Even now when I do interviews, people say, 'Why is he trying to sound like a black man?' They should hear my dad talk, he makes Bob Marley sound like the Queen.

When I turned pro, team-mates would assume I was part of the traditional 'rugby family', meaning middle-class and white. Not that I can blame them, because people see what they see, and the bare facts are that I went to a private school and had light skin. And anyway, I don't care if people think I'm white, black or purple.

I'd never say you shouldn't be proud of where you came from and who you are, but if the most important thing is the colour of your skin, your sexuality, or whatever, and that's how you choose to define yourself, you're voluntarily separating yourself from wider society and adding to division.

I understand why people feel they have to identify as something, because it makes them feel wanted, safe, like they're part of a tribe. But as soon as you say, 'I'm part of this group, and this group defines me', you've put yourself in a box and closed yourself off to other experiences and viewpoints. Essentially, you're saying, 'This is how I am and this is how I must be for the rest of my time on earth.' Plus, your happiness is dependent on being validated by other people. And if other people don't see you as you do, that's going to upset and depress you.

Figuring out who you are might be a long, painful journey or a short, painless one, but not knowing when you set out is part of the beauty. And if you fix on an identity, decide that because you're black or white, straight or gay, you must think and act in a certain way, you'll never take the first step.

I don't believe in God, as in a man with a white beard to worship, but I do believe in God, the creator of the universe. And because the same material makes up everything in the universe, the universe is everyone, and God is in everyone. Ultimately, I believe we are more than our body and mind, so why get bogged down in something as limiting and divisive as identity?

Having said all that, it's just nice to have a few brothers around the place, and we're continuing to tear the place up. Even when we're under par, as against Worcester in March, we still score six tries and 40 points.

Kurtley doesn't appear until 2017 because of an injury, but when he finally gets himself fit, he's an absolute menace. Meanwhile, Willie le Roux, who's been shifted to the wing to make way for Kurtley at full-back, is back in the kind of form that saw him nominated for world player of the year in 2014.

Willie's been out of favour with South Africa for a while, and is extremely strong-willed, like most players from that part of the world. But we worked together on positioning, timing and tempo, and different ways to get the ball into Willie's hands as often as possible. South Africa just wanted him to go at 100 mph for 80 minutes, but by easing off the gas and scanning more, he's getting himself into more try-scoring and try-assisting positions.

We play Leinster in the quarter-finals of the European Champions Cup, and they've got Lanny as a coach. Journalists are talking about it being a rehearsal for the upcoming Lions tour to New Zealand. My old Wasps coach Warren Gatland is in charge, but Andy Farrell is defence coach, so I'm not sure if there's any truth in that rumour. But even if there is, I don't get much time to practise my lines.

I spend all week in the physio room, because of a hamstring tweak, and the first time I train is at Friday's team run. Meanwhile, Lee Blackett has introduced a couple of new line-out plays, thinking they'll catch Leinster on the hop. Like most trick plays, they work in training but rarely in a game.

We have to be on it, because Leinster are bastards to play in Dublin. They're always so well drilled because they know each other so well. Most of those guys are seasoned internationals who have been playing with each other since they were kids, so their united front is genuine, not manufactured. They play more like a street gang than a team, and will fight for each other to the death.

Rugby players are never 100 per cent fit, and I've played lots of games almost on one leg. But that's far harder to do against a side as good as Leinster. As it turns out, we lose 32–17, I'm accused of getting stage fright and I don't get picked for the Lions, or England's tour of Argentina.

Owen's going to New Zealand with the Lions, but Eddie's opted for Ford, Lozowski and Piers Francis, who has been playing for the Blues in Auckland and has never played in the Premiership. It's as if Eddie's scouring the planet to find fly-halves to pick instead of me.

We thump Saracens to finish top of our group table and earn a home play-off semi-final against Leicester, and our tally of 86 tries is a record for a season. In a hard-fought, cagey affair against the Tigers, Josh Bassett, on for Kurtley, goes over in the corner with two minutes left and we win by a point.

Our opponents in the final are Exeter, who we've beaten and drawn with this season. They beat European champions Saracens in the semis and are a decent outfit, solid and united, but I think we should put them away. Then Dai starts changing things.

Dai hasn't coached much all year or said a great deal in meetings. He's like Eddie, he lets the coaches under him do the day-to-day grunt. But now Dai's all over everything. He's calling meetings about meetings, and they're getting longer and longer, with more and more talking. Watching this unfold, I just get the feeling he's getting more anxious, which is rubbing off on the team.

It's the opposite to Shaun, who might have plenty to say before a game we're expected to win, to make sure we're on it, but who melts into the background in the lead-up to a big game. Big games were never about him – it was about making things as clear as possible for his players, the people who needed to do the business. His messages would become shorter and more to the point. And on the day of the game, he'd give players little notes, highlighting one or two things to focus on. By the time we ran out on the field, we'd have tunnel vision.

It's not really like that before the final against Exeter, and we're all at sea for the first 39 minutes. We're trailing 14–3 on the stroke of half-time, when I trigger a counter-attack that leads to a try for Jimmy Gopperth. A couple of minutes later, Wadey chips through, Elliot Daly touches down and we're suddenly leading.

When Jimmy knocks over a penalty midway through the second half, we're six points ahead. We're being battered up front but still three ahead with a minute to go, before Nathan Hughes gets penalised for sticking his hands in the ruck. Gareth Steenson slots the penalty to make it 20–20 and we head into extra-time.

The teams are still level with five minutes on the clock, but we're the ones hanging on for dear life. God knows how many phases they've had, but it's like being smashed by waves. They think they've scored but the TMO decides we've held it up. But when Matt Mullan is pinged for pulling down the resulting scrum, Steenson kicks the three points to win it with two minutes to go. We had our chances but our discipline let us down. Exeter deserved it.

While England are in Argentina and the Lions are in New Zealand, I'm trying to ride waves in Malibu. Laird makes it look as natural as walking, and maybe it is to him, because he's been doing both since he was about a year old.

There's something very humbling about surfing. I'll be wobbling about on the board and a seven-year-old will glide past me. I'll think, *Fuck this, I can't have a little kid showing me up*, before smashing head-first into the water.

I'll fight tooth and nail to get beyond the waves, and I've got cramp and a belly full of salt water before one comes along that looks good enough to catch. Then when I try to ride it, I'm not relaxed enough, I topple sideways and have to start all over again. As with anything in life, it takes a lot of effort to get into a promising position, but getting into a promising position is only half of it. That's where the art comes in. However, if you're resilient enough to keep trying, you'll master it in the end. It will be you and your board riding the movement of the Earth, and all that effort will be a hazy memory.

My body's starting to creak a bit – groin, lower back, Achilles – so I feel entitled not to do stuff in training that I think is going to exacerbate things.

Every club I've been at since Wasps first time around, I've told the coaches I can't do down and ups, because they give me a tight back. So whenever we're asked to do them, I'll do little hops instead. Most of my team-mates laugh, but some coaches don't like it, think I'm being different for the sake of it. That's why Hask sometimes says to me, 'Danny, mate, just fucking do it', because he can see it's pissing coaches off. He's only trying to look after me, but I'm not doing something that's not in my best interests.

If down and ups made me a better rugby player, I'd be doing a thousand a day. But they don't, they make me a worse one. A tight back makes my groin hurt, which means I can't kick properly. So it's actually just me looking after my body, so I can be at my best for the team. And anyway, I go above and beyond in other areas. I drive miles to see Kevin and Margot, I spend hours trying to understand the game better. I'm just not going to do stuff for show.

Most people haven't played sport for a living, but I get the impression pro rugby isn't much different to an office environment. Every office has characters who always turn up early and leave late, as well as attend every meeting, sit at the front and contribute. And every office has characters who are sometimes late and sometimes duck out early, as well as skip meetings and stay quiet when they do show up. And we all know who's more likely to get on at the company. Never mind that their work is humdrum and nothing they say at meetings makes much sense. Never mind that the characters who are sometimes late, sometimes duck out early and aren't into meetings actually do far more valuable work. Bosses want an easy life, so they go by box-ticking.

Rugby is so backwards when it comes to tailoring to individual needs, because it's so caught up in this idea that allowing players to do their own thing undermines team unity. Dai reckons that if we don't run a certain number of kilometres during the week we won't run enough at the weekend. That makes no sense. We're healthy athletes, we don't need to be running a set number of kilometres to be fit for a game. Plus, Saracens scrum-half Richard Wigglesworth tells me he runs about 12 km a week, which is less than half as much as us.

Why would you have Wadey slogging up and down for hours when he's all about bursts of pace? I know why, because it's how Dai has always done things, and therefore how he thinks things should always be done, even though all that running has given loads of the speed athletes in the squad Achilles tendonitis, including me.

I injure my knee in the defeat by Harlequins and they reckon I'll be out for up to three months. The docs think I need an operation, but Kevin suggests otherwise. And because there's nothing Kevin doesn't know about bodies, I believe him.

Some of the people I train with in Malibu are regular fasters, and they're functioning at the top of their game, physically, mentally and spiritually. So I phone Laird and ask him to explain the science of fasting to me.

Laird says that when you're injured, your body requires a lot of energy to mend whatever has gone wrong. But when you eat, a lot of energy is diverted to digesting food (fasting can also improve clarity). So I fall into a routine of eating a big, healthy meal at 6 p.m., followed by another biggish one at 8 or 9, and then not eating anything until the following day at 6 p.m. again. I'm working my nuts off with Kevin in between, and the only things I drink are water, black coffee and Berocca.

One day, while I'm recovering, I read an article by Matthew Syed in the *Times*, in which he lays into me and Gavin Henson. He calls us wasted talents, says we're arrogant, fixated on partying and celebrity, and that we don't take training seriously. Ironically, Matthew writes books, some of which I've read and enjoyed, and here he is judging a couple of books by their covers.

It's nice that some of my old team-mates defend me on social media, including Wasps hooker Rob Webber and England prop David Flatman, but the article is so damning and ill-informed that I want to have a word with Matthew myself. So I send him a message – something along the lines of, 'You've heard a few whispers and think that's me?' – and we arrange to meet.

Over coffee, I tell him about the lengths I've been to since I was a schoolboy. All the extra training I've done with Margot, paying for Kevin out of my own pocket, all the extra hours I've spent on the training ground, honing my craft, all the months spent working my arse off to recover from injuries. To his credit, Matthew takes it on board and writes a follow-up article which corrects some of his previous assumptions, and we become friends after that.

I wish more journalists were able to admit they got things wrong. As it is, they think that once they've written something, they have to stand by it, come what may, as if it's a commandment chiselled in stone. That's probably why journalists never ask to chat with me outside of a controlled press conference environment, maybe over lunch or dinner. They're worried it will force them to re-appraise all the negative things they've written about me and start challenging the prevailing view, which is never comfortable.

Have you ever seen two people arguing on Twitter, when one side is digging themselves deeper and deeper into a hole, and their arguments are becoming more and more ludicrous, because they simply cannot handle being proved wrong in public? That's not strength, that's weakness.

Only by questioning your own opinions, however sincerely held, can you hope to grow as a person and keep moving forwards. And only by swallowing your pride and examining all sides of a story can you hope to draw the right conclusions.

22

HOW IT'S GOT TO GO

I'm back in action a month ahead of schedule. When I say 'schedule', I mean the doctor's, not mine or Kevin's. I don't see any articles praising my efforts to return early, but I don't expect to.

While I was injured, we lost three out of five, so Dai calls a big meeting and starts shouting, 'We need to get fucking gain line!' I say, 'What do you mean, we need to get gain line? How do you want us to do it?' Dai looks like he wants to kill me, but I'm thinking, *If it was that simple, everyone would just get the ball, run hard and get gain line. Maybe try coaching us, Dai.*

In the end, Lee Blackett tweaks the attacking system that has worked so well, based on something he's seen another team do, and we're no longer creating a numerical advantage. Everyone suddenly seems hesitant, as if they're playing in a fog. But after a couple of games back in the team, we start to turn things around and look on target for a play-off place.

I've only signed for two years, so we've started talks about extending my contract. At least I thought we had.

One day, I say to my agent, 'Have you heard anything from Dai?' and my agent says he gets the feeling they're leading us on. After we hammer Gloucester on 23 December, my agent tells me Wasps have signed All Blacks fly-half Lima Sopoaga. So the whole time Dai was making me wait, he was negotiating with someone else.

The following week, I say to Dai, 'You've just made a huge mistake, mate. I've watched Lima play and he's got a good skillset, but he doesn't run games like I do.' Dai starts chuntering away, and I say, 'Don't get in my way for the rest of the season.'

Because Dai is big and imposing, he can tell most people what to do and they'll listen, no questions asked. So it's clear as day that Dai wants to get rid of me because he hates that I've got such an influence over the team.

I like Dai as a bloke, it's important for me to say that. He's a good family man with a great sense of humour, but he hates that I comment on his coaching methods and do my own thing. But, with all due respect, Dai was a prop. What do props know about rugby that isn't head down and grafting? How can they possibly see things from the perspective of a fly-half, who has to know a bit about every position on the field and where they need to be in relation to me?

I'm not putting my destiny, and that of my team's, in the hands of someone who doesn't understand the game, which is something I learned a long time ago, during my first season at Sale. If something's not right, and is negatively affecting outcomes, I'm going to say so. The first, second and third time is never confrontational, but if you keep ignoring me, I'll eventually say, 'We're not doing it like that anymore, this is how it's got to go.'

I finish the season on fire and offers start coming in from other clubs, including in France and Japan. One Japanese club offers me 50 grand a game and I seriously think I'm going to accept. Then they find out I've got a drink-drive conviction, which scuppers the whole thing. I consider taking time out from the game, but then I think, *Hang on a minute, there's an England tour to South Africa in the summer and it's the World Cup next year. Get to the end of the season and decide based on whether Eddie picks you or not.*

It's not looking very likely when he overlooks me again for the 2018 Six Nations. He picks Quins fly-half Marcus Smith instead, and Stephen Jones comes out with a good quote in the *Times*: 'Smith isn't as good as Cipriani was at 18, let alone now.' England don't exactly set the world alight and lose their last three games, including to Scotland for the first time in 10 years.

After my final home game for Wasps, a 36–29 win over Northampton in which I set up a couple of tries, the media are on Eddie's back again, telling him he can ignore me no longer. Perhaps it helps that he's in the stands and sees it with his own eyes, because when he announces his squad a few days later, I'm in it. What are the newspaper headlines? 'JONES TELLS CIPRIANI: STEP OUT OF LINE AND YOU ARE GOING HOME', or variations thereof.

The same day, four Premiership teams contact my agent wanting to sign me. Quins director of rugby Paul Gustard sends me a photoshopped picture of me in their kit. Most of the offers are slightly more than Wasps are paying me but miles away from what French clubs are promising. Meanwhile, Gloucester say they can only afford to pay me £175,000, but that they'll let me do things my way. And if I do the business in the first season, they promise, they'll overpay me in subsequent seasons to even things up.

I wonder if their offer has got anything to do with the Wasps-Gloucester game just before Christmas, on the day I found out about Sopoaga's signing. There had been a story in the papers about their head coach Johan Ackerman and his son Ruan getting into a fight in a Cheltenham nightclub, and they were getting loads of grief in the press and on social media. So before the game, I jogged over and said, 'Listen, don't worry about what people are saying, it'll blow over soon. It's been happening my whole career. Anyway, nice to meet you.' Then we took Gloucester apart for 80 minutes.

I look at all the squads and think, *I know I'm at the peak of my powers and could go to France for serious money. And I know Gloucester are paying well under the odds – I was on more money as a teenager at Wasps. But they suit me best*. I can do good things with that team. And if I do good things, maybe I'll make it to the World Cup in 2019. Fuck the money, I'm going there.

When the news breaks that I'm leaving Wasps for Gloucester, there's the predictable reaction in the papers and on social media, mostly along the lines of, 'Cipriani's off again, can't stay at a club for more than a couple of years, his coaches and team-mates clearly think he's a pain in the backside.'

Times rugby writer Owen Slot, who's always got something negative to say about me, says team-mates 'have encouraged him to change but too many times have well-meaning words fallen on deaf ears'. Frankly, that's bullshit.

The facts are these: Dai was wrecking players with his training methods and I was the only person to say something to his face. I respect Dai as a bloke, I really do, but he revealed his cards early, when he didn't pick me for that warm-up game against Bristol. And because of Dai, I'm having to hobble down the stairs every morning, and it takes me 30 minutes of training before I can run properly again, minus any pain.

I left Wasps first time around because I desperately needed to get out of the country, for the sake of my mental wellbeing. I left Melbourne because I wanted to get home and put myself in England contention. I left Sale because I felt I needed to be playing behind a more dominant pack. And now I'm leaving Wasps again because Dai's gone out and bought an All Black and clearly doesn't want me there, despite the fact that I've been nominated for Premiership player of the year and Wasps are third in the table.

Bless my team-mate Jack Willis, who does a joint interview with me towards the end of the season and says I'm often the last man off the training ground and always helping him with his passing and decision-making. Jack's young and innocent and just saying what he feels, and it's beautiful to hear.

* * *

We give Saracens a punch-up in the play-off semis, scoring five tries to their six, but still lose 57–33. People are always asking me why Saracens are so good, and it's impossible to look beyond their pack, which is pretty awesome.

Included in the starting XV are Mako and Billy Vunipola, Jamie George, Maro Itoje and George Kruis, all England internationals. Vincent Koch is a Springbok, and they've got more internationals on the bench, including Schalk Brits (South Africa), Will Skelton (Australia) and Juan Figallo (Argentina) (Schalk Burger, the maniac back-row from Namibia, must be injured). Other Premiership sides are lucky if they have two forwards of that calibre in their squad.

Saracens' back-line is decent, but the scrum-half box-kicks the hell out of everything, because they've crunched the numbers and worked out it's the best percentage play. They're very good at knowing when to jackal and when not to jackal at the breakdown, meaning they give away fewer penalties and always have men on their feet in defence. It's not the most exciting brand of rugby, but it wins trophies, which means other English teams are trying to replicate it, despite not having the players to play that way.

Everyone in rugby knows Saracens are cooking the books, you only have to look at how many internationals they've got in their squad, including two of the best hookers in the world in Jamie George and Schalk Brits, and how much they're supposedly signing top players for, which is often way under the odds.

But you also have to respect Saracens' culture. They have a strong identity, which everyone at the club buys into, from the owner down to the youth players. They've always had very good coaches, who are extremely knowledgeable about the game. Of course a club like Saracens will attract big players, but you've still got to get them all singing from the same hymn sheet.

Saracens' sense of harmony is just as important to the club's success as the money they spend. Yes, it's frustrating that they're clearly overspending, but it's an environment I'd like to have experienced more often in my career.

23

SOUNDS LIKE BULLSHIT

England have lost four in a row, including an embarrassing mauling by the Barbarians, so Eddie's under a bit of pressure when we arrive in South Africa. But it's still mostly Owen and George running official team meetings, as well as the mafia's clandestine splinter meetings.

On the training field, Eddie's always saying, 'Flat and fast, mate.' One time, I get the ball, skip out onto the next defender, play a pass and we break the line. Eddie says, 'No mate, flat and fast.' A couple of minutes later, George Ford runs a short ball off nine and gets touched after a couple of metres. Eddie says, 'Yeah, that's it, mate, flat and fast.' I'm thinking, *You want me to run short balls off nine in the middle of the field? We'd never do that in a game, so why are you coaching it here?*

Eddie's other favourite phrase is, 'Quick ball, mate.' I'm thinking, *Every team wants quick ball, that's a given. But not every team knows how to get it. That's the hard part.* Eddie seems to think that if we do everything crash, bang, wallop, quick ball will automatically follow, but it doesn't work like that, because there are 15 blokes on the other team trying to stop you.

When I started boxing, I'd go all out for the first two minutes of a round and be shattered for the last minute. Then my trainer told me to ease off, relax my shoulders and pick my punches. I now had more power but was using up far less energy, which is part of the art of boxing. In a similar vein, I look at South Africa, who are big, full of aggression and come at you like orcs, and think they can be picked apart defensively, if we just slow things down slightly.

But Eddie's not really into art, he's all about doing everything at 100 mph, getting a group of guys to be nuggety and tenacious. Quick, fast, quick, fast, keep firing into 'em. There's nothing joyful about Eddie's approach to rugby, which means there's no sense of excitement among the lads. It's tough and it's macho, us against the world, all geared towards getting a group to fight tooth and nail. That can get results short-term, but it's not a viable long-term strategy.

It's clear to me now that the RFU only employed him because they were having a crisis. England had just failed to progress from their group at a home World Cup, losing the RFU millions of pounds, so they went for a bloke who seemed as far away from Lanny as possible. But it's like when you have a shocking breakup and immediately hook up with someone because they seem different and exciting, but who are actually really badly suited to your needs.

A couple of the lads have misgivings about Eddie's methods, I know that from talking to them, but no-one's going to say anything to his face. Eddie's always going on about leadership, but he only thinks people are good leaders if they agree with him. Anyone who questions him is likely to be out on his ear.

I spend a lot of time with Ellis Genge and Kyle Sinckler, probably because they're from similar backgrounds to me. They're chippier than most, but they're props, all about physicality, being aggressive and smashing into things. Lads who grew up on council estates aren't supposed to be artists who see the beauty in rugby. We're not supposed to ask questions. That's not our place.

There is racism in England for sure, but classism is also rife. You only have to listen to how some rugby people talk about football to realise that: 'Look at those footballers with their flash cars, daft clothes, plastic girlfriends and naff celebrations.' And I suspect they think the same about me.

The idea that rugby is a more moral game than football is absolutely ridiculous. Forwards coaching is basically teaching players to pull the wool over the referee's eyes. Defence coaches are constantly telling players to slow the ball down, go offside, push the letter of the law. How is that any more moral than a footballer going down easily in the box? And I've never heard of a footballer gouging an opponent's eyes or biting an opponent's ear or finger.

Under Eddie, our time is micro-managed like you wouldn't believe. Every night, each player gets a printout, telling him how the following day will look until 6 or 7 p.m. We're even told when to sleep and how long for.

Eddie's brought along a stretching guru who gives classes every morning. I turn up on day one and everyone's there with their stretching bands. After a while, I think, *I wouldn't normally do this, so why am I here?*

There is room for science and innovation and striving for those marginal gains, but for me, it has to come from feel. I need to work out what's best for me, rather than working from someone else's rule book, just to fit in.

Eddie rules by fear, and you're never going to get the best out of people with that mindset. Why would a player make a decision based on what they see, which might be different and surprise the opposition, if they know Eddie's going to come down on them like a ton of bricks if it doesn't come off?

The way Eddie talks to his staff makes me wince. I'm told that at one meeting, a member of the backroom staff had his hood up and Eddie said to him, 'Mate, what the fuck have you come as today?' The guy replied, 'What do you mean?' And Eddie put him away with, 'Mate, don't fucking speak again.'

The next day, Eddie hands this guy a bag and says, 'Here you go, mate, some steak for you and the missus. Sorry about yesterday.' When the guy gets home, he tells his partner they're having steak. But when he opens the bag, it's actually sausages. Then he gets a text from Eddie: 'Mate, you're a fucking sausage, not worthy of steak yet.' That sort of stuff can be quite funny, but the high turnover rate of Eddie's backroom staff tells you it's not a healthy regime.

* * *

I'm not in the squad for the first Test in Johannesburg. We're leading 24–3 after 20 minutes, before conceding five tries and losing 42–39. Eddie promotes me to the bench for the second Test in Bloemfontein. The Boks are in full control when I get a run out with 15 minutes to go, and while I make a few things happen, we end up losing 23–12, making it six defeats on the spin.

When Eddie is asked about my cameo, he replies, 'Danny was one of the reserves that came on and they didn't do the job they needed.'

Eddie is trying to come across as cool, but he's clearly rattled, and that's seeping into his players. Ben Youngs storms out of a post-match interview, a couple of the lads are caught swearing at fans, and I'm not in the least bit surprised. If we were led by a wise, strong character, do you think players would be behaving like that? Of course not.

On the Monday, Eddie approaches me with a worried look on his face. 'Danny,' he says, 'have you flown a girl out here? That's what journalists are telling me, and they're gonna do a story.' I tell Eddie the truth, that I haven't flown anyone to South Africa, but I've got a pretty good idea what's going on. It can't be a coincidence that just before my first start in 10 years, the tabloids have been circling again, disrupting my return.

A girl I slept with has been telling me for ages that the papers are going to do a story on us. Being naïve, I thought she was being harassed. But now she's posted a picture of our team hotel on Instagram, suggesting she's there. I don't know if she posted the picture of her own accord and the

Mail and the *Sun* picked up on it, or whether the *Mail* and the *Sun* paid her to post it. Either way, they seem to print negative stories about me whenever I'm close to being selected by England, so it feels deliberate and malicious. And now here I am again, having to convince the boss that it's a pack of lies.

Eddie believes me, thank God, and picks me to start the third Test in Cape Town. 'Go do the business, mate,' he says. I reply, 'Okay, yeah, I will.'

It's my first Test start for 10 years and I'm sure I'm going to make a difference, like I'm always sure I'm going to make a difference. It's not exactly my kind of conditions – 'Biblical' is how one journalist describes the downpour at Newlands – but we just do what's needed. Ben Youngs mostly box kicks, meaning I don't get the ball much. But I make my tackles and chase my kicks, and when the chance comes to impose myself on the game, I take it.

When I receive the ball with nine minutes to go, I scan, see the space and execute, all in a split second. I don't have time to think, *Is this the right thing to do?*, I'm acting on well-practised instinct. When the ball leaves my foot, I think I've overdone it, but Jonny May, who's like shit off a shovel, reaches the ball first and dots it down just before it dribbles out of play.

We end up winning 25–10 to give the tour a veneer of respectability. But sitting in the changing room afterwards, it doesn't feel like we're a band of brothers, it feels like 23 blokes who have just completed individual missions.

My only real act of bonding is a photo with my old

Wasps mate Willie le Roux, who's back in the South Africa team, just as I said he would be.

Only later does it occur to me, I might have just helped save Eddie's job …

It's the final day of Gloucester's pre-season tour to Jersey and my first proper drinking session with the lads. As you know by now, I like to do my thing for team harmony, so every time my team-mates sink a pint, I sink a double rum and coke.

Things almost go horribly wrong before we've left the hotel. Deontay Wilder, the world heavyweight champion, is staying at the same place (Carl Frampton is fighting on the same show as Tyson Fury in Belfast at the weekend and is in Jersey to see Gloucester play Ulster), and me and a few other lads get chatting to Wilder and his crew in the lobby. We're getting on great, and I'm already quite drunk, so I decide to throw a Drake lyric his way: 'Yeah, I'm light skinned, but I'm still a dark n**** …'

When I'm in America, all my black friends refer to me as a light-skinned nigger – in other words, 'He may not look like it, but he's one of us' – but as soon as the words leave my mouth, I realise Deontay has no idea who I am. And he could split my jaw seven ways. Thank God, he eventually breaks into a grin and says, 'Man, I knew there was something different about you …'

It's all fine until we get to a nightclub, I try to bring a couple of drinks outside and a security guard puts his hands on me. 'No, no, no,' he says, 'you can't take drinks outside,' and I reply, 'Alright then, and neck both of them.'

We're trying to get our captain Willi Heinz into the club, but there are three or four security guards blocking the door. After a bit of back and forth, I lean across and yank one of their ties, which turns out to be a clip-on and comes off. There's a bit of a furore, before I walk off with the tie in my pocket. And a few minutes later I hear, 'Nee Naw, Nee Naw', before two police cars pull up and four coppers jump out.

One of them says, 'We believe you've been causing a disturbance', before grabbing my hand and putting it behind me. When his mate grabs my other hand, I throw them both off and shout, 'Why the fuck am I being arrested?' Then I have a moment of clarity – *you can't act like that towards the police* – and let them cuff me.

As they're bundling me into the car, I'm screaming at them to loosen the cuffs, because I've got pins and needles shooting through my wrists. And I'm screaming at them all the way to the station, 'You're a bunch of fucking idiots!'

People say, well, if the police arrest you, you should just accept it. But they haven't even told me why. They stick me in a cell and when I've slept off the booze, I don't touch the food they give me and meditate for eight hours straight.

I'm in the cell for two nights, because they reckon I'm a flight risk. When they read me my charges, they include assaulting a female police officer, despite the fact the two coppers I shrugged off were men. It gets ridiculous – 'If you admit to these two charges, we'll drop the others' – but there's no way I'm admitting to anything I didn't do. Resisting arrest? Fair enough, I suppose I did, but only because I didn't know why I was being arrested. And I didn't push or hit anyone, let alone a woman.

I pay the £2,000 fine, apologise for my behaviour and try to move on, but the media aren't going to let that happen. They make it sound like it was the Gunfight at the OK Corral. Then the *Sun* does a story claiming I said, 'These wrists are golden, loosen the cuffs!' To borrow a quote from *Apocalypse Now*, the bullshit is piling up so fast I need wings to stay above it.

Gloucester tell me they have to fine me, for appearances' sake, but then the RFU decide to charge me with bringing the game into disrepute. What the hell has it got to do with them? They didn't charge Manu Tuilagi when he was convicted of assaulting two policewomen. In fact, they've never charged anyone for a non-rugby incident. And do you know who's guiltiest of bringing the game of rugby into disrepute? The RFU, because they've been letting down the English game for years.

24

BEGGARS BELIEF

I escape with a rap on the knuckles from the RFU, but who knows what's being said about me behind closed doors. Never mind. One thing I am is resilient.

Some people still seem to think I'm a weak character, but nothing could be further from the truth. For years, I didn't think about the impact Dad leaving England had on me, or the fact I couldn't rely on Mum, but that was some heavy, resilience-building stuff. Luckily, I always had sport as an escape – my highest passion, what made my heart sing. I spent almost every waking hour playing sport and being loved for it by my friends. And when I wasn't playing, I was that naughty kid who put soap on the floor in the changing room showers, to make people slip everywhere. God, we laughed so hard at that.

I've overcome a lot through my rugby career: being placed on a pedestal before being toppled when I was still just a kid; a career-threatening injury; a deluge of lies and exaggerations from the press; being judged by a hoodwinked public; having the door slammed in my face by a succession of England coaches.

I've now realised that while I need to examine those feelings of abandonment, rejection and victimhood, in order to have any chance of healing, burying them for so long served a purpose, because it was the only way I could keep moving forwards. But let's be honest, nicking a bouncer's tie isn't exactly the crime of the century, despite the hysterical reaction to it.

I keep thinking about Wayne Rooney and the time the papers said he'd visited prostitutes. Most people would have wanted the ground to swallow them up, but he shrugged it off, won man of the match in the next two games he played, and all the negative headlines promptly disappeared. I hope that if I start the season well with Gloucester, the same will happen with me.

Whenever I join a new club, I always get the sense that people don't know what to make of me. I can tell from the way they behave that they're trying to suss me out: Is he an arrogant prick? Is he a team man? Is he someone I should be seen to be friends with? But from the moment I turn up at Gloucester, I'm bang on it, from laying out cones to laying down systems.

Gloucester haven't finished in the play-off places for almost a decade, and were seventh last season, their best finish since 2013. But I reckon this group of players can do great things, if only they start believing in themselves.

Every day, I'm working with different individuals, building up their confidence, improving their skills, getting them to understand where they fit into the system. It's not as if I'm ranting and raving at them on the training field, it's more short conversations, highlighting various bits and pieces.

I'm sure some of my team-mates are taken aback by my intensity, and I'm sure some of them think I'm a bit mad. But I do have a lighter side and join in with some of the changing room banter. And soon team-mates are saying, 'You're nothing like I thought you'd be.' I suppose they've learned that just because someone doesn't play the game, that doesn't necessarily mean he's not a team man.

Funnily enough, the thing that made me feel most accepted is when I got banged up in Jersey. When I got on the team bus to go home, someone put Akon's 'Locked Up' on the stereo and they all started singing along, 'They won't let me out! They won't let me out!' No-one was tut-tutting, everyone was cool with it. I remember one of our second-rows, Ed Slater, putting his arm around me and telling me not to worry about it.

Johan Ackerman is very prescriptive: 'If you hit here, and have a ruck there, they'll overfold over here, then space will open up over there ...' Thinking two or three phases ahead has its place, but it can't be your overall ethos, because rugby is a chaotic game, in which things hardly ever go to plan.

How many times have you heard someone say, 'You have to earn the right to go wide?' But it's just a cliché that's been passed down the generations. You can't play the game based on managing risk, and you can't not do something because it doesn't fit in with a diagram a coach drew on a whiteboard. If the space is there, you have to be prepared as a team to use it.

Coaches have said to me, 'Your way isn't going to work, because not everyone sees things like you.' But what I do isn't magic, like card tricks aren't magic. Ballplaying is teachable, as is more esoteric stuff like drawing out defences and manipulating space. A lot of it is just empowering players, allowing them to make their own decisions, and sometimes fail, within game scenarios.

Concussion is a big talking point in rugby at the moment, and rightly so, because players are getting dementia as young men. But changing the tackle height and reducing the number of games aren't the only solutions.

We need younger coaches with more progressive ideas, people who approach training with more finesse and emotional intelligence. Too much rugby training is a grind, something you've just got to get through rather than something that's enjoyable and inspiring. It's imposing men barking orders like sergeant majors and players feeling like squaddies, trying to do everything with a big weight on their shoulders. It's tough and macho and doing everything with a stiff upper lip. As a result, I often find myself managing my energy for game days, instead of feeling energised and fizzing with enthusiasm.

I have played in teams where the coaching was more thoughtful, with the emphasis on technique. But at Sale, if the coaches decided we hadn't been physical enough on the Saturday, Tuesday's training session would be brutal. We'd play six against six in a grid, and it would just be people running at each other. No-one emerges from an archaic, unrealistic session like that a better player. Plus,

I've seen lots of players get injured doing those kinds of drills.

If a boxing trainer told a fighter to have wars in sparring, people would think he was out of his mind. In modern boxing, they understand that training is as much about preserving the body as toughening the body up. They also understand that the best way not to get concussed is not to get hit.

If rugby training was more about evasion than contact – creating and exploiting space, making players agile and evasive rather than stiff and lumbering, like mummies – players wouldn't get so many whacks on the head, with the bonus that the game would be a lot easier on the eye. But coaching players to have the skillset to make the right decisions, depending on the defensive set-up, takes time and patience and a level of understanding that most coaches simply don't possess.

The fly-half has a huge role to play in terms of managing a team, but you can never have too many ballplayers. Problem is, too many English coaches have the attitude, 'You're big and strong, so just run straight and hard.' Whereas they should be saying, 'Yes, you're big and strong, but if you work on your passing game, you'll be an even bigger handful for defenders.'

The perfect example is All Black great Ma'a Nonu. When he started out, he was very direct. But over the years, he developed his passing and kicking game, which meant his running game became so much more effective, because defenders didn't know what he was going to do and were sitting off him.

I don't understand sportspeople who are happy to tread water. That's why I find Eddie's coaching so baffling, because none of it is to do with individual player improvement. If a player is big and strong, Eddie will just tell them to run like the clappers, and not much else. He's got this big reputation as a rugby sage, but his methods lack nuance.

People will say, 'An England coach can't improve a player in the short time he has with him, it's just a case of slotting them into a system.' I don't agree. In a three-week camp, there's loads a coach can do.

If you're a strong, courageous coach, you'll tap into a player's energy and help him grow. You'll give little pieces of technical advice, open a player's mind to different perspectives, empower him to try things, make the game feel easier. If a coach comes from a place of love and wisdom, you'll want to hear whatever hard truths he tells you. That's how it was with Shaun.

Shaun could be harsh, but only because he wanted me to improve. On the flip side, shouting at someone for doing the 'wrong' thing isn't loving or wise, not if it makes a player feel small and uncomfortable, it's just shouting at someone. If a coach does that to me, that's when we have a problem, that's when conflict arises.

At Gloucester, there's a prop called Fraser Balmain who's got great hands but is reluctant to use them, because coaches have drilled it into him down the years, 'Don't make mistakes.' I can see the fear in Fraser when he's trying to make a pass, so I say to him, 'Mate, you're just passing a ball, it's no big deal. And if you practise it enough, there won't be any risk to it.'

We've got a talented centre called Mark Atkinson, who's got a great short passing game and excellent footwork at the line, but who keeps throwing long miss passes. I say to him, 'Why did you do that? What did you see?' He replies, 'There was space out there.' He's right, there was, but the defence was on the slide, meaning we ended up with a ruck on the touchline, which is the easiest position on the field to defend from.

I say to Mark, 'Rather than throwing three long miss passes a game, focus on your short passing game. I promise you, when you stop looking for those Hollywood passes, it will suddenly become obvious when one is actually on.' It's just what Shaun used to teach me, about taking responsibility for your actions on a rugby field, which naturally leads to fewer mistakes.

I persuade our scrum-half Willi Heinz to run less and pass more. 'Willi,' I say, 'I know England want you to be a running nine. But the more you run for the sake of it, the less quick ball we get. Whereas if you only run when something is on, they'll think you're a running nine, even though you're not actually running as much.' I get on great with Willi, so he's very receptive.

I'm man of the match in our first two games of the season, a win against Northampton and a draw with Bath. Eat your heart out, Wayne Rooney.

People are raving about the no-look miss pass that sets up Matt Banahan's late try at the Rec, but I did something similar the week before against Saints. I've been honing my decision-making skills for years, but this season at

Gloucester feels like a step up. I'm able to stay in the zone for longer periods than previously, and the group is in tune with what I'm trying to do.

A rugby field is my safe space, my natural environment. Every time I pull that cherry and white shirt on, I feel like a super-hero changing into costume, before setting out on a mission. This is what I've been put here to do.

I'm assuming Eddie saw that pass against Bath because he was sitting in the stands. But a few days after another win against Bristol, which Eddie also watches in person, he announces his squad for the autumn internationals. You know the script by now.

The *Guardian* calls my omission from the England squad baffling, the *Independent* calls it madness, the *Sun* calls it bizarre and brutal, not so much an axing as an assassination. Brian O'Driscoll says it beggars belief. In the *Times*, Stephen Jones says that Eddie must be on a different planet.

Eddie says it's got nothing to do with what happened in Jersey, is 100 per cent based on form and that I'm probably the fourth best fly-half in the country.

Because it makes so little sense, I'm starting to get a bit wrapped up in conspiracy theory. Maybe I shouldn't have made that pass against Bath, because it's given Eddie another excuse – 'He's just a highlights player.' But I'm not out there throwing 30-metre, no-look passes for the hell of it, like those footballers you get who can do loads of tricks but rarely set anything up. I take accountability for my actions on a rugby field, so if I throw what appears to be a mad pass, I'm doing it because I've worked on it and know it's the right thing to do.

Eddie keeps banging on about my lack of work-rate off the ball, but who picks a fly-half based on their work-rate off the ball? As it stands, I'm the best decision-maker in the country, maybe the world, and as Eddie's seen with his own eyes, I only need one chance to win a game. It's not an honest evaluation of what's happening. I'm even starting to wonder if shadowy figures at the RFU are leaning on him.

Eddie calls me and says I need to be better at going to the line. I say, 'Eddie, I'm the best in the world at going to the line.' If Eddie doesn't want to pick me, cool. But just be honest about it. Say you want to play the game a certain way and I don't fit in with it.

In a press conference, Eddie says that phone call was like splitting up with a girl, which sounds quite terminal. Making a joke about dropping me is also really disrespectful (not least because it gives the *Sun* an excuse to run the headline, 'I JUST CALLED TO SAY I AXED YOU'). Most journalists and ex-players seem to think my goose is cooked. But I'm not giving up. The only way I can make the World Cup is to keep doing what I'm doing, but even better.

A week later, I win Premiership player of the month. Besides the proper award, the lads in the TV studio present me with a trophy of a pair of golden wrists. I laugh along through gritted teeth. I know it's only harmless banter, but everything coming out of the media just seems so personal, even when they're on my side.

The following day, we play Wasps in Coventry. I'm revved up for that game, really want to rub Dai's nose in it. And that's what happens. I score 15 points in an easy win and spark one of the tries of the season. I could have run the last 10 metres and scored myself but dropped the ball onto my foot and set up scrum-half Ben Vellacott to score next to the posts. After what went on at Wasps, it feels delicious.

ED SLATER

When I heard that Gloucester had signed Danny, my first thought was, *Bad decision*.

I'd come through the Leicester system, which encouraged certain kinds of characters and behaviours. Leicester players were no-nonsense blokes, and those were the kind of people I admired. As far as I was concerned, that was how to be successful, and anyone who was different I didn't relate to.

I didn't know Danny very well, but I'd read lots about him and heard bits and pieces, as had everyone at the club. Overall, there was a mixture of excitement and uncertainty. We all knew what a good player Danny was, but he had this celebrity status – London, nightclubs, modelling, women – so some of us worried he'd bring some of that off-field chaos and be disruptive.

When I heard Danny's version of his arrest in Jersey, I didn't know what to think. Then I heard what happened from a couple of people who were with him and realised he'd done nothing wrong beyond nicking a bouncer's tie.

It was actually a good start to our relationship, because I thought, *Maybe the things I've read and judged him on aren't true. Maybe he is treated more harshly than the rest of us*. The media storm that followed reinforced that opinion. I said to him, 'Danny, don't worry about it. Nobody's angry, we're all behind you, let's just put it behind us and get on with things.'

When we got down to training, some of the guys were taken aback by his intensity. They'd expected a maverick, someone only worried about himself, but he improved everything and revolutionised how we played.

I was blown away by Danny's depth of understanding. His rugby IQ was streets ahead of everybody else's and he changed how I saw the game. And it wasn't just me, he improved us all. Mark Atkinson was doing okay before Danny turned up, but Danny took him to a different level. The fact that Mark played for England wasn't solely because of Danny, but he had a lot to do with it.

Danny challenged and argued with people, which I loved. I knew that for the team to be successful, we needed characters like that. I could also see how it made Danny quite difficult to manage. Coaches have egos, and they're meant to be in charge, so their authority needs to be respected. But Danny had such an inner belief in his ability and understanding of the game that he felt it was his place to openly question how things were being done.

Johan loved playing an open, expansive game, which suited Danny. But they saw the game slightly differently – Danny was very technical, Johan was more of a big vision person – and because they were both big personalities, it ended up in a bit of a power struggle. There were lots of good times, but there were some tense, difficult moments along the way.

I understood Danny's frustrations, why he felt he deserved more of a say in training, because he was running the team on game day. But I tried to get him to understand that the team listened to him, respected him, and backed him. That was the most important thing, not being seen to be in charge and getting stuck in this power struggle. I think Danny took that on board. He never stopped being challenging, but he did rein things in a bit.

Could Gloucester have done what they did without Danny? We were a team on the up before he arrived, and we'd have done well anyway. But he was brilliant that first season, and improved lots of his team-mates, so I'd say he was the difference between us finishing in the top four or not.

I'll never forget some of the moments of magic he produced – the whipped long pass to Charlie Sharples, out of nowhere, on his debut against Northampton; the comeback win against Bath at Kingsholm; the return against Northampton at Franklin's Gardens, one of my favourite ever games, when he put on an absolute masterclass and got the whole team firing.

But however good Danny was for Gloucester, it was never going to work with England under Eddie Jones. There was no way on God's earth that Eddie was going to allow Danny to challenge him, and I'm guessing that Eddie felt that unless Danny was the out and out number one, he'd do more harm than good. I also wonder if Danny would have been happy playing second fiddle for England, because he's got such strong views. To have to play back-up to a game-plan that didn't suit him wouldn't have been easy.

That said, Danny should have been used more by England over the years. But that would have required bravery, at a time when rugby was becoming more risk averse. Coaches are led by stats and numbers, so there's lots of kicking, lots of playing for territory, lots of chat about pressure. You don't have to be the best rugby player in the world to play that kind of game, which is why some coaches viewed Danny as a luxury they could do without.

We had an amazing 12 months with Danny on the field, and I got to know him well off it. We liked deep and meaningful conversations, during which I found out more about what made him tick. He had this image as a party animal, but he was a quiet, shy, considerate bloke. I count myself lucky to have seen that side of him. If more people had, coaches included, maybe they'd have understood him a bit better and not judged him so quickly.

I was worried about Danny during his second season, because he came across as quite unstable. I asked him a couple of times if he was okay, but I don't think he felt comfortable talking to me about that stuff at that time. I got the impression there weren't many people he felt comfortable talking to.

The talk he gave to the team after Caroline Flack's passing only made me worry more. He looked and sounded like he was completely overwhelmed, and that's when it became a difficult situation for everyone at the club.

He never lost the respect of his team-mates, but that intensity on the field dropped off a little bit. And suddenly there were a couple of questionable characters at the club who wanted to exploit the situation for their own advantage, as well as a couple of others who wanted to batter him. Meanwhile, there were a lot of us stuck in the middle, just wanting to support him, but not knowing how.

I'd never been around somebody going through the kinds of problems Danny was – somebody who was questioning everything about their life – so I didn't know how things would turn out for him. I did, however, fear the worst. But he's in such a good place now, which is great to see.

After I was diagnosed with motor neurone disease in the summer of 2022, Danny was one of the first people to get in touch. And a couple of weeks later, he drove up to see me. And it wasn't a one-off, he's visited a few times since, and we message each other often. Ignore all that tabloid nonsense, Danny's just a really lovely guy, thoughtful, generous and kind.

Once upon a time, when I was still young and a little bit naïve, I thought there was only one way to be a good person. But Danny made me a lot more accepting of different personalities. I take a lot of pleasure from being wrong in my initial assessment of Danny. I wish more people knew the real him.

25

HERE FOR A REASON

I was feeling great in training, and performing well in games, but I was still spending hours on my own, making the same mistakes. I knew that I didn't want to be making them, which was progress, but I couldn't get out of the loop.

Friends in Malibu advised me to try mushrooms, said they might help sort out the chaos in my mind, so I experimented with them in the off-season. I haven't told anyone back in England because people will get the wrong idea. Mushrooms aren't on the banned list, but people will think I've gone all weird.

I dabbled with cocaine in the past, but have cut back on the Tramadol, and for the most part I won't go near anything man-made. However, anything from the earth is cool with me. The way I see it, these things have been part of certain cultures for thousands of years, cultures that are much more in tune with nature than ours is. That suggests they're here for a reason.

I tried crystalised toad in America, which was a deep experience, and I'd like to give ayahuasca a go. Ayahuasca is a brew made from an Amazonian plant, which you drink as part of a day-long ceremony. I'm told it opens lots of different doors in the mind, but I'll probably have to go to Peru to try it, because it's not the sort of thing you can buy from a geezer at Croydon bus station.

The famous psychoanalyst Carl Jung believed everyone has a shadow self, associated with negative emotions, that they suppress from childhood. Only by confronting our shadow can we ever really know ourselves and hope to untangle all those negative emotions that have been holding us back. Mushrooms contain psilocybin, which turns all your senses up a little. Images are brighter, sounds are clearer, thoughts are sharper. I've seen it described as a waking dream, which works well. And after a micro-dose, I'll think about something traumatic from my childhood and see it from a different perspective. It will feel softer, less intense, and I'll have more compassion for anyone else involved. Plus, I'll keep hold of that new perspective even after the sensory effects of the mushrooms have worn off.

When I do take Tramadol, it's to numb the mind and body, and I still distract myself with women, although far less frequently. But there's nothing frivolous about mushrooms, it's an integral part of the quest I'm on to better myself.

In micro-dosing mushrooms, I'm only doing what humans have been doing since they developed the capacity for thought, namely trying to figure out what the hell is going on. *What are we? Where did we come from? Why are we here?* Mushrooms don't give me definitive answers, they just create different possibilities. They make me feel like I'm going with the flow of the universe, instead of constantly trying to swim against it, which is utterly futile. I know that to be the case, because I tried to do it for far too long.

I've watched my mum and dad avoid their issues and it's not been pretty. It feels like alcohol is playing its part, and when Dad came to stay for a month, he'd disappear for hours and turn up at night wasted. We didn't talk about it, but I think he just felt safe down the pub. And I assume he was trying to blank out a lot of regret.

One day he tells me that Chelsea wanted to sign me when I was 10. 'Are you kidding me?' I say, 'why didn't you tell me?' Dad says, 'Because I wanted you to have a full experience of life.' Damn it, I could see myself playing up front at Stamford Bridge. But unlike Dad, I don't have regrets. I'm starting to see that everything happens as it's meant to, which means I'm better equipped to handle whatever may be. On Christmas Day, I'm invited to the Heinz house for dinner with Mum. Willi and his family are kind, beautiful souls. We eat and drink and enjoy ourselves, but as the day progresses Mum gets more belligerent and it feels like she's belittling me at every turn. Willi's wife says I'm great with her kids but Mum can only laugh. 'Danny? Not my Danny?' The next day, I wake up, make Mum breakfast and ask her to leave. She doesn't remember much of the day or what she said, but it feels like the last straw. On my way to training, Willi's wife calls to tell me that her 12-year-old daughter couldn't understand why Mum wasn't proud of me. It really hit home that day. I realised that I needed to create a safe space for myself.

* * *

If any of my team-mates had a problem with my intensity when I first arrived at Gloucester, I can safely say that at least some of them have changed their tune.

We're playing some superb rugby, we're winning, and Kingsholm's Shed Army are raising the roof at homes games. And if there's one thing that makes sport enjoyable, it's your efforts being well received by your team's fans. It also helps that some of the lads, including Willi Heinz, have been called up by England. Willi's kind enough to thank me for my help in one of his interviews.

Everything's going swimmingly, until February, when director of rugby Dave Humphreys offers me a contract extension way under what he promised. I say to him, 'This isn't what we agreed. You've underpaid me this season, which I'm fine with, but you were supposed to make up for it.' I was fuming.

Before our home game against Exeter, I see Dave walking towards us and shout, 'Fucking get back inside, I don't want you out here!' That's not the way to deal with it, but I feel betrayed, shafted. I've played out of my skin, dragged them up by the scruff of their neck, exactly what I said I was going to do, and now it feels like they lured me there on false pretences.

A few days later, Dai calls me out of the blue and says he wants to meet for a chat. Wasps have been very patchy this season. They've still got most of the same players as when I was there, but Lima Sopoaga hasn't worked out like Dai thought he would. Lima, who's on big money, is getting a lot of stick and I feel for him. He thought he was just coming in to play 10, not realising that in New Zealand he's surrounded by people who instinctively know how to play, but in England rugby is far less intuitive.

I'm interested in what Dai's got to say, so I agree to meet him in some depressing motorway hotel, like where Alan Partridge lived. The first thing Dai says to me is, 'Danny, I got it wrong. I now know you weren't the disruptive one. I now know you held the team together. He then starts pointing the finger at another player, who's signed for another club and Dai feels betrayed by.'

Dai promises that if I come back, I can run the team and do my own training. But the whole time I'm thinking, *I'm not sure he's being sincere. I think he's just panicking because Wasps keep getting battered.*

I tell Dai I'll think about it, then he walks me to my car. Before I can get in, he gives me a big hug. Part of me respects that Dai appears to have revised his opinion of me, and I do still have a strong emotional attachment to Wasps. But I wonder if he's really willing to do things differently, and I'm still irritated by what happened.

If Dai had been more open to conversations, I wouldn't be earning less than half as much money as I was last year. I wouldn't have had to up sticks and move home again. And there would be far fewer people saying I'm trouble, a bad apple, an arsehole no team can trust. So no, I won't be re-joining Wasps.

* * *

Despite the success we're having at Gloucester, Johan still wants things done exactly his way.

I'm having weekly meetings with him, trying to make him understand what I'm doing and why I'm doing it. He'll say, 'Why do we keep talking about the same things?' I'll reply, 'Because we need to get better!'

Johan's a good man overall, but like most coaches I've played under, he's stubborn. Some nights, I'll be sat on my sofa thinking, *Why won't Johan listen? This sport is ridiculous!* Then again, maybe it's all these barriers I keep coming up against that make me so driven.

Eddie's still not seeing me. Well, maybe he is, but he's certainly not recognising me for who I am and what I can do, because I'm not in his Six Nations squad. The usual offers come in from French clubs, but I still haven't given up hope of playing in the World Cup. And after some tough negotiations, I agree a new deal with Gloucester and focus on our title push.

We're 17 points down against Bath at Kingsholm, before I get the boys in a huddle under the sticks just before half-time. I tell them what we need to focus on and how things are going to pan out after the break, and the next time we have the ball, I throw a no-look pass to our tight-head prop and he goes over for a try. We score three more tries in the second half, win 27–23, and clinch a place in the play-offs for the first time in eight years. Job done.

Louis Rees-Zammit makes his debut that day, and he's just turned 18. Louis is seriously quick, a little bit special, and I've loved watching him come through. To the coaches' credit, they've given him some rope and allowed him to find out who he is. You always hear stories about old pros knocking young players down a peg or two, as if it's the natural way of things. But the way I see it, if you don't try to learn from the kids coming through, you're standing still.

The following month, I'm voted Premiership players' player of the year. And a few days before our play-off semi against Saracens, I'm named Premiership player of the season. I also win the rugby writers' award. So there you have it: Eddie thinks I'm the fourth best 10 in England, pretty much everyone else thinks I'm the best player in English rugby, in any position.

It's nice to feel loved but I can't enjoy it. I'm numb after months of back and forth with Johan, I've got a play-off semi-final coming up, I'm desperate to play for England in the World Cup. When I look in the mirror, I see a mess.

As before last year's play-off semi, I'm confident we can beat Saracens until the Monday before the game, when Johan starts meddling, just like Dai did.

Because it's a big occasion and he wants to be the man who masterminded victory over the mighty Saracens, he introduces complex new line-out plays, ignoring the fact that the beauty of our starter plays is their simplicity. Why would you have players learning new plays the week of a semi-final anyway? You want to play a big game without thinking and just doing.

I know the Shaun Edwards way – downplaying the game's importance, keeping a low profile and making the messages as simple as possible – sounds scary. But a coach should trust that adrenaline will naturally flow and the desire that's carried the team that far will manifest itself when it matters most. Instead, Johan keeps going on about the game's magnitude and how good the opposition are. And suddenly, he's presiding over an anxious group.

Here's another good story to illustrate how Shaun dealt with big occasions. When I was 17 and Wasps reached the Anglo-Welsh Cup final, Shaun brought me and Dom Waldouck into the changing room, to give us a taste. And an hour or so before kick-off, he went through the whole team, giving a little profile of each player.

'Here, lads, we've got Eoin Reddan, one of the best decision-making scrum-halves I've ever seen. We've got Paul Sackey and Tom Voyce on the wings, two slippery buggers who are almost impossible to tackle. We've got Mark van Gisbergen, whose goal-kicking is metronomic.' And so on.

After Shaun had run through all the replacements, he moved onto the guys who weren't in the squad, finishing with Rob Hoadley. Rob, who everyone called 'Dave', worked hard in training and put himself about in games, but would readily admit he didn't have much of an X-factor. However, he was really into his fashion and always wore funky outfits. So Shaun finished with, 'And last but not least there's Dave, best-dressed man in the Premiership.'

That was just perfect timing. Everyone had been getting more and more pumped – *Fucking hell, if Shaun thinks we're great, we must be* – but when he dropped that joke, everyone cracked up. Suddenly, the atmosphere was light and relaxed. And the joke didn't have a victim, because

Rob was well aware of his place in the team and he and Shaun had a great relationship.

Inevitably, the media bill the game as a duel between me and Owen Farrell, and my final audition for a World Cup place. That's not how I see it, I just want to win the game. Unfortunately, Saracens are a very well-drilled outfit. We score an early try and have more good moments, but Johan's late tweaks have confused the team and we end up losing 44–19.

26

WHEN YOU NEEDED SOMETHING DIFFERENT

I head to Malibu, where I stay with the NBA player Joakim Noah, who I've been training with for the last four summers. I spend five weeks training like Rocky Balboa – running on the beach, ice baths, pulling logs, underwater weights, working on agility. The only thing Joakim doesn't have me doing is chasing chickens, but it's refreshing training with someone with such drive outside the rugby bubble.

Eddie calls me up for his preliminary World Cup squad and we all gather at the Lensbury hotel in Teddington. Most of the boys congratulate me on my awards – 'Fuckin' hell, mate, some season' – and the papers are full of articles by ex-players saying Eddie has to take me to Japan. But I'm acutely aware that it doesn't matter how many people say nice things about me. It all comes down to one man's opinion, as shaped by members of his mafia.

Eddie's usually okay with me in person, even cracks the odd joke, the kind of stuff that makes you think, *Did he really just say that?* But this time he's on me straightaway. Just my presence seems to irritate him.

I'm creating line breaks in training, but Eddie never comments on them. Instead, he keeps telling me what I'm not doing that he thinks I should be. I'm thinking, *Were you watching what I did a few minutes ago? I created a try. Why are you focusing on the negatives?*

It feels like Eddie's going out of his way to disrespect and belittle me. Bear in mind, I've had Willie le Roux and his Springbok team-mates facetiming me after games, wanting to hear my views. Why don't I get that kind of respect in England? I'm not asking for special treatment, just a few encouraging words every now and again.

After a week, Eddie takes me aside and says, 'Mate, you're not fit enough. You need to go away for a week and train on your own.' I'm dumbfounded. I've just spent a month in Malibu working my nuts off. The World Cup doesn't start for nine weeks, isn't that the point of this training camp? And anyway, I'm at the same level as the rest of the boys in the fitness tests we've done. None of this is real, none of this is honest.

When I tell Margot I'm coming to see her, she can't get her head around it either. But if Eddie wants me to get fitter, she'll do whatever she can. I train with Margot every day for a week before Eddie calls me back to Bristol. But when the bulk of the squad flies off to an acclimatisation camp in Italy, I'm one of 10 or so left behind. We do bits and bobs, but I look around at the other lads, who are all young, peripheral players, and I know the door is finally shut.

Actually, it's worse than that. For four years, I've been obsessed with playing for England at the World Cup and

I've given it absolutely everything. But it suddenly occurs to me that all my hopes and dreams were based on an illusion. I was banging my head against a door that didn't even exist.

If they'd given me even a handful of starts on the bounce, and licence to run the team, I could have got a beautiful tune from that England team. Instead, I've been strung along, made to look a mug, verging on delusional. Why didn't Eddie yank the Band-Aid off years ago, instead of peeling it off slowly? It feels cruel, almost sadistic.

When he finally calls me to deliver the coup de grâce – 'You're fitter, mate, but you're not going any further' – it really does feel like a death, as if I'm fading from the picture. I can't really hear him, and I don't say a word.

I've heard people say Martin Johnson, Stuart Lancaster and Eddie Jones can't all have been wrong, whatever Shaun Edwards or Brian Ashton thought of me. But I tried it both ways – not playing the game and playing the game – and neither worked out for me. Besides, it's not as simple as who was right and who was wrong, because sport is ultimately about results.

Maybe if I'd kept my head down and been more yes sir, no sir, Johnno would have persevered with me. But a deeply traditional rugby man like Johnno was never going to want an opinionated kid like me involved. And look at what happened at the 2011 World Cup, England were an absolute disaster.

Lanny was given the job far too early and wasn't really in charge anyway. I never had a chance, what with how they wanted to play and the influence of Andy and Owen. But why not be honest? If you thought I was too much of a risk, just say so.

For years, people have been asking why England don't play with freedom and creativity. And general sports fans, who only really watch international rugby, probably assumed I was scraping a living in the Premiership, a shadow of the kid who dazzled against Ireland at Twickenham in 2008. But I've been playing like that week in, week out since my second season at Sale. Or maybe they assume I never stopped being the horrible bloke the press made me out to be.

I'm not outwardly emotional, but I'm broken and empty. I turned water into wine with Gloucester, and the blokes Eddie's picked voted me the best player in England just a couple of months ago. I feel like a character in a computer game with a fatal glitch. I've completed every level, collected everything I was supposed to, but the game keeps telling me I can't win.

Gloucester want me to come back in straightaway, but I tell them I need some time off. Johan tells me I can have a week, I tell him I want five. He's not happy, but I don't give a shit, because my head has completely gone.

I head back out to Malibu, where I train and party with Joakim, Blake and Devin Booker. But I can't shift the thought that Eddie's going to call me up at some point. It happened to Stephen Donald in 2011, when the All Blacks lost three fly-halves through injury and Donald kicked the winning penalty in the final.

Alas, there's no fairy tale for me. On the morning of my first Premiership game of the season against Sale, England play New Zealand in the semi-finals. And they're phenomenal. Eddie gets his game-plan just right, his pack dominates, his defence is watertight, and England win quite comfortably.

The final against South Africa is on my 32nd birthday. I bring myself to watch it, along with the rest of the Gloucester lads, before our game against Leicester. I'm not going to lie to you, part of me won't be too disappointed if the Springboks win.

International rugby should be about preparing a team for all eventualities, whether it be the need to kick long, kick and chase, attack through the short side, attack through the middle, or all the above.

But with South Africa demolishing England up front, Eddie doesn't appear to have a plan B, let alone a plan C or D. You can almost see the players thinking, *Shit, this isn't going how we expected it to. What do we do?* Meanwhile, I'm sitting there thinking, *Just when you needed something different …*

JONNY WILKINSON

When Danny came into the England team, I felt intimidated. I was struggling with injuries at the time, trying to stay in control, trying to survive. And here was someone with a very different energy, who had the breath of youth, who was exploring, creative, free, all things I was envious of and resistant to.

I remember Danny saying something along the lines of, *It must be nice being you*, and me thinking, *I wish I could be a bit more like him*.

When Danny replaced me for the Six Nations game against Ireland in 2008, I watched his performance and thought, *Here's a guy who's better for the team than me. He's brought freshness and enthusiasm, he's brought Twickenham back to life*. His spontaneity reminded me of what I was like, back when I was 18 or 19. And I started to understand that I'd got a bit lost.

After the game, a journalist asked what I thought of Danny's performance, and I said I was learning from him. I meant it, I was. Yes, he was seven years younger than me, but he was taking the game in a new direction.

I was too into myself to see things as a fight between us, but I get why the media took the opportunity to play us against each other. When you're young, you want to be seen and heard for who you really are. But the media don't want to find out who you really are, they're only interested in creating narratives, even if they're not accurate.

That said, there were differences between me and Danny. I still felt able to run free for my club side Newcastle, even though we weren't winning many games. But for England, being the saviour was how I'd come to express myself, so my game was based on managing events, being in control, being the safe, steadying influence. Meanwhile, Danny was looser, tried things. Off the field, I was seen as more typically rugby, because I said the right things in the right accent. Meanwhile, Danny seemed like an outsider, a maverick.

When I was playing, it was the guys who did miraculous things I found most inspiring, especially if they were on my team. But that didn't necessarily mean they were the best players. Coaches have bigger decisions to make: Who are we playing against? What are the conditions? How do we need to play to win? Team selection usually comes down to a couple of opinions, and most coaches favour players who do damn fine stuff a lot of the time over players who do miraculous stuff some of the time. And they don't chop and change for specific games because they have long-term plans.

I know from the early part of my England career (and the middle part, when I spent a lot of time injured) that only if you're able to string a few games together will you connect with your team-mates, create a sense of purpose and inevitability, and build momentum. And Danny was never given that chance.

Should he have played the game a bit better, as in said and done things differently off the field? Well, I'd say that being authentic to yourself is the only thing that really matters, and that any time you spend not being authentic is taking you in the wrong direction.

People will read that and think, *That's easy for you to say, you won a World Cup*. But while I had plenty of success in my rugby career, a lot of inaccurate things were written and said about me (I didn't suffer as badly as Danny, but still), and there were times when I wasn't really me.

I played for Newcastle for 13 years, and after winning the Premiership in 1998 and the Tetley's Bitter Cup in 2001, we won nothing. In fact, we spent most of the next eight years battling relegation. But if I was to make my own highlights reel, most of the clips would come from games I played for Newcastle in that period. There were only a few thousand people watching, and not many people were reading about us in the papers. But I engaged so fully and played so well. Things didn't always go right, but I was being me.

For a long time, Danny regretted not being allowed to do what he could do for England. But I played for England however many times and I still have issues with the way certain things panned out. If you're a competitive beast, whatever happens is never going to be enough.

I say to Danny, 'I'm not interested in what level someone's playing at, I'm interested in watching players express their genius, which is beautiful to watch.' Sometimes that genius will get you picked for England, sometimes it won't. And while I've got no doubt that Danny was capable of performing at the highest level, it's more important that he expressed himself at all times.

A few years back, I did some work with Marcus Smith. When I asked him how the game against Gloucester went at the weekend, he said, 'You should have seen this sick thing Danny did ...' I was looking at Marcus thinking, *That's what it's all about*. It doesn't matter if Danny's doing it in a white shirt or a red and white shirt, it matters that he's inspiring people. And Danny's done that almost everywhere he's been, revealed his genius, made people sit back and say, 'Fair play to the bloke.' Not many people can do that.

Knowing Danny as I do now, I see things very differently from when he first arrived on the scene. Now, I realise it was pointless wanting to be more like Danny, because it was just how I was, the only thing I could be. But we've both discovered that while we are very different on the surface, we've always been after the same thing, just come at it from different angles.

When we meet, neither of us is trying to prove anything. It's not about competition or comparison, it's about sharing. That's where the bond comes from. When Danny tells me some of the stuff he faced, I think, *Wow, people should just be amazed he got on the field, let alone achieved what he did*.

Once upon a time, rugby seemed like such a big thing. But now it seems like peanuts compared to what me and Danny are exploring now. Our lives were never without their challenges, but we've reached a stage where we're asking to be challenged, in order that our journeys can continue.

Danny is loving working out what's happening inside of him, as opposed to trying to correct everything on the outside. As a result, he's translating the effortless power he demonstrated on the rugby field to life in general. Sometimes, I listen to him and think, *Jeez, this stage of Danny's life is going to be more powerful than his playing career, and that was powerful enough*.

Listening to someone talk about stuff they've done can be fun, but I'm more fascinated by people who are always evolving and living in the present. That's why people who live comfortable lives often aren't particularly inspiring, while someone like Danny has got an awful lot to teach people.

Life should be about transformation, and the change in Danny has been immense. The scary thing is, his rate of change seems to be accelerating, as it is for me. Every time I meet him, I think, *Blimey, he's moved on again*. And he's not even trying to become anything, he's just allowing it to happen.

Maybe we should be thankful for all the challenges he faced, because these are the fruits.

27

REVEALING THE REAL ME

In rugby, being fully seen means playing for England, so none of the awards I won in my first season at Gloucester made me particularly happy.

Worse, having worked so hard to make things work at Gloucester, it doesn't feel like my team anymore. When I turn up to pre-season, Johan's changed things up completely, so everything suddenly feels alien to me, and there isn't the same excitement and energy in the group.

A few days before our home game against Saracens, they get hit with a 35-point deduction for salary cap breaches. I'm far more surprised that Premiership Rugby actually punished them, although they did it in a very rugby union manner. When rugby league's Melbourne Storm got done for salary cap breaches, the trophies they'd won while cheating were taken away.

I'm not angry, but I am irritated. I think back to when I was at Wasps first time around and they had to start selling players off, to stay within the salary cap. If that group of players had stayed together, Wasps could have created a dynasty. To be fair, other clubs could say the same.

A few weeks after Saracens are punished, Eddie releases his memoirs. According to the papers, he mentions me more times than any other player, which is odd considering he's hardly ever spoken to me. Apparently, Eddie says I'm incapable of changing, which is pure projection on his part.

Ironically, given Eddie's Japanese heritage, *Kaizen*, which is Japanese for 'continuous improvement', has been at the forefront of Blackie's teachings over the years, and I've never stopped studying the game of rugby and adapting. Whereas once I was a young, exuberant, explosive ballplayer, I'm now older and wiser, and I take pride in transforming an entire group of players.

I'm happy someone like Eddie didn't pick me, because it must mean he didn't see anything of me in him, which can only be a good thing. I hope he's cool and has a good life, but carrying around a chip that size on your shoulder must be exhausting, and he doesn't strike me as a peaceful or happy man. Not soon after, Ben Te'o, a rugby league legend who successfully crossed codes playing for Leinster, Worcester and England, writes an article about his best cross-code starting thirteen. In it, he shares that he's 'never seen a ball player like (Cipriani)'. Having played alongside some top players across both codes this feels like high praise from Ben, but unfortunately it's too little too late.

Johan's waving the conductor's baton and I feel like I'm playing a broken piano, while surrounded by people playing instruments with strings missing.

We lose five on the spin in November and December, before stopping the rot with a win against Connacht in the Champions Cup. There's a social media debate over whether I meant my cross-kick for Louis Rees-Zammit's try, but of course I meant it! I've seen Aussie rugby league great Cooper Cronk do it, and I did it against Harlequins last season.

If you square your body up and shape to chip kick, the other team's open winger assumes it's going to be dinked over the line and starts dropping back. So if you hit it cross-field, he'll be out of position and one of your own backs will be able to run onto the ball with acres of space in front of him.

Some people can't conceive of an English fly-half doing something like that deliberately. They think that because most English fly-halves would have punted the ball down the field in that situation, that's the only option. But I've always abided by that Bruce Lee quote: 'Absorb what is useful, discard what is useless, and add what is specifically your own.'

If players only ever did what their coaches told them to, the game would never evolve. But there aren't many free-thinking fly-halves around, blokes who are willing to say, 'Never mind what I'm supposed to do, I'm gonna find out different ways of doing things.' That's why I enjoy Finn Russell's approach to the game. He's a guy with a very high skillset who has the courage to execute. But even he's been in and out of the Scotland team, because head coach Gregor Townsend, ironically a creative 10 himself, has never fully trusted him.

Our form improves either side of Christmas, but I'm still struggling for motivation. Then I tear my calf playing against Montpellier in the Champions Cup.

While I'm out of action, I'm speaking a lot to Caroline Flack, the TV presenter. We've got mutual friends and dated last year. We managed to keep our relationship secret for about a month, before being papped kissing in her car. Neither of us wanted the scrutiny that would accompany a 'celebrity' relationship, so we decided we'd be better off as friends instead.

Caroline has been tabloid fodder for years, not only because of her TV work but also because she's been in a few celebrity relationships, including with Prince Harry and Harry Styles. Last December, she was charged with assaulting her current boyfriend, and she's due to stand trial in March.

Like they did with me, the media and public are judging Caroline on snippets of her life, rather than the full picture. And because she's a celebrity, a lot of people think she should just lie down and take it. I struggle to understand that attitude. Everyone on this planet has to deal with suffering, everyone makes mistakes, so why aren't people more understanding?

Caroline is a beautiful soul, so it's hard to fathom that people are so happy to revel in her misfortune and discomfort. I can only think that judging someone else, and imagining themselves to be morally superior, makes them feel slightly better. But that feeling is illusory, and it won't last long.

When I tell Caroline about the various scrapes I've been

in and the media harassment, she says to me, 'How come you're so positive? How come you're not burdened by the way they treated you?' I tell her I haven't always been so positive and unburdened. But I also try to assure her the tabloids and social media vultures will forget soon enough, as they did with me, and that good times will come again.

It's a Friday evening and I'm in the changing room before our game against Exeter. My phone rings and it's Caroline's number, but I can't answer just before kick-off. So I send her a quick message instead: 'Can't speak, about to play a game, speak to you after. Everything alright?'

After the game, I check my phone and Caroline hasn't replied. I message her again, still nothing. First thing next morning, I try again – still nothing – and this time I notice my messages are only getting one tick, which means she isn't opening them. Later that day, I find out Caroline has taken her own life.

I've never cried so much. All I can think is, *Why didn't I read the signs? And why didn't I answer her call? It was only a game of fucking rugby.*

I could have told her everything was going to be okay, that things were going to change, that one day she'd look back and wonder how she was ever so unhappy. Instead, she made an impulsive decision based on how she felt in that moment. I know how she felt, because I've been there, so deep in a hole that I couldn't see past the end of my nose, let alone a future. I thought I was going to be in that hole forever, and the only way out was to end things.

I make it to work on Monday and Johan starts yacking in the meeting. I usually let it slide when he's talking shit about rugby, but this time I say, 'Coach, you're wrong.' His son Ruan pipes up with, 'Danny, you've always got something to say', and I go frothing-at-the-mouth mad.

Johan pulls me into his office and things get a bit heated. But after things have calmed down, Johan says he wants to say sorry to me in front of the group and I tell him I want to say a few words to the boys as well.

We re-join the rest of the lads and Johan apologises, before I stand at the front of the room and a lifetime of trauma comes flooding out: everything I went through growing up, all the shit I've faced from the media, how I've spent years not wanting to look over my shoulder, for fear of being seen and judged, all my dingiest secrets, all the things I'm ashamed of. I talk about stuff I've never discussed with anyone, including the time I felt so low I wanted to kill myself.

It must be harrowing for the lads because I'm a sobbing, snotty, shaking mess. After I'm done, some of the older boys are a bit standoffish, as you'd expect. I'm not normally emotional, and a bloke bearing his soul is a rare sight in rugby. They probably think I'm having a breakdown. Thinking about it, I am, in that I'm breaking down years of things I've held on to. Revealing my wounds feels like the only way to free myself.

The younger lads, some of whom have already sent me beautiful messages, are more generous with their hugs. A few of them tell me I'm brave, but I don't see it like that. My pain, sadness and grief made it something I had to do, rather than a choice. There was no other way, I'd kept it in for too long.

I barely sleep or eat for the next few days and the weight is falling off me. But I still go to work every day and tell Johan I want to play at the weekend, to show people that you've got to keep going, whatever happens.

On the Wednesday, I tell my agent I'm going to do a video, because there's stuff I need to say. I'm not sure my agent knows what I'm going on about, but I get on the phone to a cameraman I know, and he comes down to Cheltenham. I'm not sure what's going to come out when he turns his camera on, I just know I want to get things off my chest, only this time publicly.

When I finally stutter into life, I explain how kind and loving Caroline was, and what unkindness had done to her in return. I describe everything I've felt embarrassed and shameful about, and explain that it was embarrassment and shame that killed Caroline. And I talk about how it's okay to be vulnerable. I couldn't save Caroline, but I do it for her. I also do it to save myself, and I do it for anyone thinking that taking their own life might be the solution.

It's maybe not the best career move, because being truthful and vulnerable can make people feel uncomfortable. But there are things in life that are more important than career moves. I wish Caroline was still with us, and everyone who knew her will miss her terribly, but the pain, sadness and grief I feel at her passing has made me embrace my vulnerabilities even closer.

After playing in the game against London Irish, I'm given a few days off. A friend who knows a thing or two about grief advises me to turn off my phone and TV, sit in silence for 48 hours and write down whatever comes to me. For the next two days, I scribble pages and pages of notes, scrunching them up and throwing them away as I go. It's not about keeping or analysing, it's about getting everything out, as fast as you can. When I emerge, I feel a lot lighter.

28

MESSY AND BEAUTIFUL

A couple of weeks before Caroline's passing, my mate Ed, the guy who paid me a visit when I was at my lowest ebb and trying to buy a gun – got married in South Africa.

I was one of his best men, and he said some beautiful things about me in his speech. I could feel real love in his words, which made me quite emotional.

When the party started, I spent time sitting on my own, watching Ed dancing with his beautiful wife Olivia, their friends dancing on tables, his parents and stepparents all having fun together. I thought back to when we were kids, when Ed's parents split up and found new partners, and how difficult that was for him. But now it felt like forgiveness and joy had washed that all away. Later, I took Ed aside and said, 'Mate, you've really made me believe in love today, for the first time in my life.' And I started tearing up.

Rewind to 5 January and I'm out for dinner with some friends. There's a woman there I've never met before, called Victoria Rose, and I find her very intriguing. She's beautiful and has real presence. At the same time, she's one of the first women I've met that I don't see eye to eye with.

Usually when I talk to women, I'm playing a role, a game, only revealing enough to get that familiar buzz. But Victoria can see straight through me. She's happy to call me out on my bullshit. She asks questions and disagrees with my answers. She winds me up and presses my buttons. I wouldn't say I enjoy it, but it's certainly more stimulating than I'm used to, just as a fiendishly difficult puzzle is more stimulating than a wordsearch.

A couple of weeks after our first meeting, we hook up. We carry on chatting but don't have time to see each other again before Covid hits. In early March, they decide to suspend the Premiership and I head off to Malibu for a week, to sort my head out. When lockdown kicks in, I get stuck there.

The whole of America has lost the plot, but I'm able to carry on almost as normal. I feel pretty flat, but I can run, have my saunas and my ice baths, read books, listen to podcasts, practise deep breathing. I keep having to tell Gloucester I can't get a flight home, and I end up living in Malibu for three months.

I'm still out there when Victoria tells me she's pregnant. I'm unsure about it, but say to her, 'I will support you in whatever decision you make.'

When she decides to keep the baby, I'm so excited. Even at 18 I wanted to be a dad, despite the way I was carrying on with women. And although me and Victoria aren't planning to be in a relationship, I suggest it's our duty to get to know each other properly, to be true, and to be the best parents we can.

We start chatting all the time on the phone. The early

conversations last a couple of hours, but they soon end up lasting five or six. I hold nothing back, and it's the first time I've ever been fully truthful with a woman. It's intense, it's profound, and through it all, Victoria makes me feel comfortable.

After two weeks, and hours and hours of conversation, I realise I've fallen in love with this incredible woman. And when I finally return home, Victoria collects me from the airport, we go straight to my house in Cheltenham and spend every day together for the next two months, having only met four or five times before that.

Victoria is a stunning woman, but it's not just her beauty that dazzles me, it's also her heart and soul. She's worldly wise, wildly intelligent and compassionate. I think she's the first woman who has genuinely cared for me.

Victoria knows what I'm thinking from small changes in my facial expressions. She knows when I'm sad and trying to look happy, or when I'm frustrated and trying to look calm. She knows when I'm lying about anything. Meanwhile, I can see Victoria becoming softer and freer with every passing day.

Have I been in love with women in the past? Since meeting Victoria, I'm pretty sure I haven't. I've met lots of great women, and had some great experiences, but none of them made me feel safe or comfortable enough to reveal the real me. With Victoria, it's different. I can reveal all my ugly truths, my shadow, my darkness, and still be accepted and loved, which is what real love is.

It would be mad to say that someone you meet and don't get on with might be the perfect partner for you. But hundreds of times I've felt that metaphorical 'spark', followed by a couple of weeks feeling lovestruck, before realising that spark wasn't going to take flame. With Victoria, it's different.

Me and Victoria have intense conversations about my parents, my relationships with women, my bullshit and manipulating, my rugby career, my relationships with coaches, team-mates, the media and the public, my depression, my reliance on painkillers. At times, she must feel like Sigmund Freud. But by opening up and letting Victoria in, I'm learning more about myself. Victoria makes me want to be a better man. Although you can't just want to be a better person for someone else, you have to do it for yourself.

Victoria says to me sometimes, 'Danny, you're so gullible.' She's right, and maybe that stems from the fact that people have lied to me about so much.

I don't think I'll ever know all the ins and outs of my mum's story, but what I've learned from the rough outline is that true resilience isn't just ploughing on and never facing up to bad things, it's trying to make sense of them as they happen, getting them off your chest, making them a thing of the past, like brushing off layers of rust. Mum has spent her life running with a huge weight on her shoulders and she deserves to be free of it. It's tough knowing there is nothing I can do but be there for her.

Then there are the messages my dad used to send me, asking for money. The first one nice and long, the second shorter, the third something along the lines of, 'Dan, I'm struggling. I can't afford food, I can't afford to pay the rent ...' For years, I felt like I had to keep bailing him out, because he was my dad and I loved him. But Victoria says to me one day, 'Maybe stop giving your dad money and see what happens.' I do, and the messages tail off.

Since childhood, I'd had Dad on a pedestal, because he was my best friend, the person I had most fun with, my escape. Finally seeing the truth was difficult, but the one thing that always trumps truth, however ugly, is love and forgiveness. I still love Dad, I'm still thankful for the life he's given me and the joy he's showed me. I'll always be there if he needs me.

It's not as if Victoria sits me down and teaches me to be less gullible, but because of the love and trust we've built up in a short space of time, she can tell me hard truths. That can sometimes feel uncomfortable, as it can for her. Like me, Victoria is a complex character who's been through a lot of trauma, but there's a lot of strength in two complex characters coming together, and she's slowly opening up.

We have some great times during lockdown, and I'll remember this period as messy, beautiful and life changing. I don't think Victoria would describe it as fun, although she might describe those conversations as necessary. Is she grinding things out for the sake of our baby? It's possible she was at the beginning, but I now know how quickly she flees a bad situation.

I suspect Victoria will look back and feel grateful that we had this opportunity to bring our histories, ideas and beliefs together and spend so long sifting through them, discarding things we don't need, keeping things we do. It's been the most beautiful and enjoyable challenge, with true love as the prize.

When news gets out that me and Victoria are together, women start bombarding her with stories about how horrible I was. There are also the inevitable articles in the papers, along the lines of 'STEER CLEAR OF CIPRIANI – HE'S BAD NEWS'. Most women would run a mile, and it can't be pleasant for Victoria, but she takes it all in her stride.

Victoria's got three children, and I've always wanted to be part of a big family, so when her son Kam moves in with us, I'm chuffed. I'm not sure Kam likes me much at first (he does, after all, have Google at his disposal), but as stepdads have done since time immemorial, I dig a football out, we head to the park, and we soon start making progress.

When lockdown eases, me and Victoria head to London for a weekend. I ask for the hotel room to be covered in flowers and rose petals, and when we walk in, I drop to one knee, pull out a ring and ask Victoria to marry me. She says yes.

A month or so later, Victoria loses the baby. We call him River, and his nose is just like mine, spread across his face. It's difficult to take, for both of us. But the impact our beautiful little boy has on our lives is powerful. River played a big part in freeing me, which I'm desperate to honour for the rest of my life. Because of River, I shared parts of my soul with his mum I might never have known existed. His spirit united two loving, determined individuals, opened them up and sent them on a wonderful journey of discovery.

VICTORIA CIPRIANI

The first time I heard Danny's name was in 2014. I was giving my friend's friends a lift into London, they were in the back, and they were arguing about Danny, who they were both sleeping with. But they weren't tearing each other's hair out, which I found odd, they were saying how nice he was and how much they loved him. Eventually, I turned around and said, 'Are you two girls mental?'

But I also thought, *He must have something pretty special going on for these two beautiful girls to be so besotted with him, despite him treating them with such disrespect*.

The first time I met Danny, I thought he was a bit of a wally. He wasn't boastful – 'I'm this, I'm that' – but he did have an air of arrogance.

I questioned everything he said, which unsettled him. And while I assumed he disliked me, we couldn't stop sending each other messages.

He must have spent hours writing some of his texts, because they were like essays, but I'd just reply with, 'Right' (if I say 'right' to him to this day, he looks at me with contempt). One time, he texted, 'Hello beautiful. Send me a pic.' By which he meant a naked pic.

I was astounded that women would fall for such a primitive line. I texted back, 'Does that really work? I don't know what kind of women you've been dealing with, but I'm not impressed.' He never got a picture from me.

I blocked and deleted him a few times. But there was something about him that kept me coming back. I could tell he was a compassionate soul, and I sensed his pain – a pain that was also inside me, although deeply hidden.

When I found out I was pregnant, I was distraught. I thought it was the universe stitching me up for things I'd done wrong, and for weeks I pretended it wasn't happening. Then I saw the video Danny posted, after Caroline's passing. Lots of people were saying how brave he was, but I just saw a broken man.

I waited 11 weeks to tell Danny I was pregnant, and even then it was via text. I expected him to raise the question of ending the pregnancy, but instead he said, 'Whatever decision you make, I'll support you.'

I didn't answer his calls for eight days, but eventually summoned the bravery to speak to him. That's when he started telling me about his own childhood and how he didn't want to raise a child like his parents raised him.

It was the first time he'd spoken about that to anyone, and I began to understand why he was how he was. My heart bled, and I wanted to reach out, give him the biggest hug and let him know it was all going to be okay. But I didn't for a moment think I wanted to be in a relationship with him.

Then, over the course of two weeks, during which I really started to understand Danny and his heart, we started to get excited about having the baby. And while I knew Danny had a lot of work to do, I could see what a beacon of light he was, even though he couldn't see the light himself.

One day, he sat me down and said, 'I've got all these things to tell you and you're going to hate me afterwards.' I thought it was going to be some far out, horrific stuff. But after his big reveal, I said to him, 'Danny, none of what you've told me is that bad. They're certainly not things to feel guilty about for the rest of your life. Forgive yourself, don't keep carrying it.'

When the news came out that we were in a relationship, I received thousands of messages, from many different women he'd slept with over the previous however many years. There were conversations they'd had with Danny, pictures of them in his bedroom (although Danny wasn't in any of them). But I wasn't angry or upset, I just felt sorry for the women.

I lost the baby around the same time as Danny ended up in the Priory. When I visited him for the first time with his mum (who I was meeting for the first time), I didn't recognise him, which was alarming. He fell to his knees, hung on to my waist and, between the big, heaving sobs, kept telling me to take him home and kill him. Meanwhile, his mum was telling him to sort himself out and stop seeking attention, which only added to my shock.

But that period, harrowing as it was, just brought us closer together.

It turned out that every preconception I had of Danny, based on how he'd been portrayed in the media, was wrong. I wasn't the only one. Sometimes, people would chat to Danny and say, 'You're so different to how I expected you to be', and I'd see a pang of sadness in him. That's how dangerous the media can be.

I could never understand how the man I lived with could smash people to the ground on a rugby field. He wasn't this gregarious stallion of a man, he was soft and gentle. He wasn't flashy or materialistic, he bought shirts in Zara and never wore a watch, let alone an expensive one.

Danny could be challenging if he didn't understand something, but he was never argumentative. He never raised his voice, and seldom swore in front of me. So when his friend and Gloucester team-mate Henry Trinder told me that Danny can be pretty outspoken in a rugby environment – that if he had something to say he'd say it, come what may – I was somewhat taken aback.

But Danny never told me he was unfairly treated, whatever was going on in his head. And he's over the fact he played for England less than he wanted to. Besides, I think he'll be an even better coach than he was a player, because he sees things other people don't and is a genius at improving people.

I thought I was great at badminton, but I played Danny once and he started giving me advice: 'Just relax your wrist, move your thumb to here ...' That was the best I'd ever played, but he still beat me. In fact, I've never seen anyone beat him at anything, even if he's never played it before.

When Danny's got a message to deliver, he's intense. I find it stressful at times, because I'm quite resistant, like he used to be. But the journey he's been on has made me look at myself and think, *You know what? I need to do some healing as well, because I need to live in the same place as him.*

I'm a work in progress, but we're on this journey of self-healing together, moving forward in the knowledge that while a relationship can go from harmony to disharmony, it can repair itself and return to closeness.

Most of the time, Danny just floats around looking peaceful, so I call him a spiritual zen warrior. He even has a smile on his face while he's doing the dishes. And he's got such a dry sense of humour, comes out with off-the-cuff comments that have people in stitches. He's the most kind-hearted gentleman I've ever met, a wonderful husband, stepfather, son and friend.

There's nothing he wouldn't do for my children or granddaughters, Rosie and Lily, and he only ever brings love and light to the table. Danny and I still want to have a child together, so we're continuing to explore the possibility of being parents together. He will be the most present father anyone's ever seen.

I've always thought it was telling that while Danny has lots of friends from rugby and the entertainment world, his best friends – the ones he cares about most and who care most about him – are people he's known since childhood. That's the sign of a man who never forgot where he came from.

If only his parents could see what an incredible person he is. I wish they'd tried to get to know him properly, instead of always putting themselves first. I'll never understand the dynamics at play, but I just can't imagine not speaking to or seeing my children as often as I could.

People ask me all the time, 'Are you not worried that Danny's going to cheat on you?' Maybe the unhealed version of Danny would have contemplated it, but he's a completely different person to the man I met, so I have no fear. He loves who he is now, which is heartwarming to witness, and he's in love with me. Boy, have we had to work for it, but we feel tremendously lucky to have each other.

Sometimes Danny will say to me, 'Vic, I just needed to be loved and cared for properly.' He'd been wronged and unfairly judged by so many people, when all it took was one person to take the time to discover what a beautiful person he is.

Danny calms my soul. He makes me feel loved, safe and secure beyond measure. The love he radiates created the space for me to examine my own patterns of behaviour and enabled our marriage to thrive. I respect and admire his resilience, courage and strength. Four years after we first met, every time he walks through the door, smiling his beautiful head off, my heart still skips a beat. I'm looking forward to forever.

29

HAPPY TO BE ME

Gloucester's chief exec calls six senior players in for a meeting, including me, and tells us Johan is off to Japan and that the club needs a new head coach.

He shows us the shortlist, which includes plenty of big names, and the only candidate I'd follow is George Skivington. I was in the same year as George's brother at Donhead and George and I ended up playing together at Wasps, where we became really close. George has never been a head coach before, and I'd never petition for someone to get a job simply because he's a friend. But George is honest, leads with his heart and has a knack for unifying a forward pack. Everyone agrees he's the ideal fit.

Alex King, another old Wasps team-mate, is hired as attack coach and we play some great rugby after the league restarts in August, including a seven-try drubbing of Leicester. But we still finish seventh, four places worse than last season. And when the new season gets underway a little over a month later, I don't want to be at Gloucester anymore.

I thought I'd be able to reconnect after Covid, Caroline's passing and falling in love with Victoria, but my head's just not in it. I don't feel like I can be myself on the field, which is no good for me and no good for Gloucester.

Around that time, I overdo my mushroom intake and think Victoria's trying to kill me. I'm standing at the top of some stone stairs in the garden, thinking, *The only way to escape this terrible experience is to let go*. So I put my arms out, lean back, topple over and smash my head on the edge of a step.

Victoria hears my skull crack and reckons she can hear gas coming out. She's crying hysterically because she thinks I'm dead. But a couple of minutes later, I leap off the floor, run past her and lie down on the living room floor, with a cushion under my head.

Victoria calls an ambulance, and the next thing I know, I'm surrounded by people trying to give me CPR. I'm losing a lot of blood but I won't let any of them touch me. I still think Victoria is trying to kill me, but she's the only person I want close.

I vaguely remember coming to, getting in the ambulance and arriving at the hospital, but the trip continues. I think there's a big conspiracy against me, and everyone is in on it, from Victoria all the way down to the nurses. While I'm lying in the hospital bed, doctors and nurses are constantly poking their heads around the curtain to get a look at me.

After being discharged, Victoria puts me in the Priory for a week. I barely eat and lose loads of weight. When I go for a walk in the garden, the flowers and the birds don't seem real. This goes on for five or six days.

When I finally come out of this trip, I realise that fear was driving it. The fear of not being loved, the fear of not being enough. That told me there was still plenty of buried trauma that needed unearthing and sifting through.

A couple of weeks later, I arrange a meeting with George and tell him I can't justify my wages, because my head's not in the right place, and I don't feel as if I've got a good grip of the players since Caroline's passing and my team address. 'Listen, George,' I say, 'I need to take some time away from rugby.'

George wants me to stay and fight, but also understands where I'm coming from. When news of my departure is announced, George says lots of nice things about me, and makes it clear there has been no bust-up. But that doesn't stop other people weighing in with their negative opinions.

Lawrence Dallaglio claims it was Gloucester who got rid of me, and rounds off his column thus, 'It didn't last, it never does. And at some point you've got to look at the mirror and say, "You know what, it may just be me."'

Months go by, and I still don't know if I want to play again. It's Victoria who encourages me to start making a few enquiries, because she can see my eyes light up when I talk about rugby. And eventually I conclude that there's still more for me to do in the sport.

I meet Bath director of rugby Stuart Hooper and he says all the right things, just like Dai did before I re-signed for Wasps. I'm wiser now, realise that when a coach says, 'I want you to run our attack', what he really means is, 'I want you to run my idea of attack.' But I look at Bath's squad and think that if I can get their best players in all the right places, we can do some damage.

I sign in March 2021, but it's agreed I won't play until the following season. So on 27 April, me and Victoria take the opportunity to get married.

We were supposed to tie the knot on 6 January, the day after our one-year anniversary, but Covid scuppered that. And when we finally get around to it, it's just me, Victoria, two of her friends and Kam. We've agreed it's just a legal thing, and that I'll organise a special wedding on a beach in the Caribbean or the Maldives, which is what Victoria deserves, but I'm mad proud nonetheless. I never thought I'd be married. I sometimes wondered if I'd even be alive at 33.

I've been at Bath a week when I say to the attack coach, 'I think we're missing some key fundamentals.' He replies, 'Yeah, grab the boys for five minutes after training and show them what you want them to do.'

Grab the boys for five minutes? It's got to be more than that, it's got to be a key message, it's got to be part of a philosophy, we've got to design drills around it. But after the fourth or fifth conversation with the attack coach, I realise he wants things done his way. So for the first time since I was at Wasps as a kid, I sit back and let a coach do exactly what he wants.

It feels so alien to me at first, but it's strangely peaceful. I don't have any conflict, I just go into work every day, train and go home, like most people.

Bath finished seventh in the league in 2020–21, but Stuart is bullish about the new season in the press, saying we're targeting a play-off place and maybe even a trophy. I'm not sure why, because there's an obvious disconnect between Stuart and his head coach Neal Hatley.

Neal was England's scrum coach under Eddie, and I don't think he ever wanted me at Bath. He certainly hasn't made me feel very welcome. Plus, he's South African, as is the attack coach, so he wants us to play in the Springbok style, with the emphasis on box kicking, chasing and hitting rucks hard.

But while it's a simple and seemingly safe way of playing, it's based on fear. And you can't just say, South Africa are great, that's how we need to play. Sport doesn't work like that. If you want to emulate how another team plays, you have to understand exactly how and why they do what they do.

Victoria is excited about moving to Bath, until she turns up to a pre-season game and another player's missus says to her, 'My boyfriend's the hotshot around here, not yours.' It's like she's walked onto the set of a bad American high school movie.

There's a different vibe at Bath to any club I've been at before. All the boys seem decent, but they don't seem to have much faith in the coaching group. It's more a case of turning up to training every day and putting their best foot forward, while not really buying into things. As a result, I sense it's going to be a bad season. But it's miles worse than I ever could have imagined.

My debut doesn't go well – we lose by a point to Sale and I have to go off after a whack on the head, which means I miss our defeats by Newcastle and Bristol. I finally make my home debut against Saracens, and it's a complete nightmare. They score 10 tries and we lose 71–17, Bath's biggest ever defeat.

Someone close to Neal tells Victoria that he doesn't want me around the place, but he continues to be lovely to my face. I'm relegated to the bench for the games against Quins and Wasps, but we lose those as well.

The guy who takes my place at fly-half is Orlando Bailey, who I've really taken a liking to. He's talented and intelligent, but quite soft-natured and slightly lacking in confidence. I think, *I'm not gonna have any influence over the team, but maybe I can have some influence over Orlando and the other youngsters*. But the defeats keep coming, whether it's me or Orlando playing at 10. They're not narrow defeats either – Leicester, Northampton and Gloucester all put 40 points on us.

We end up losing our first 12 games, which is mystifying on the face of it. We do have a bit of a horror show in terms of injuries, but look at some of the players we've got: Wales number eight Taulupe Faletau, England back-row Sam Underhill, plus Jonathan Joseph, Anthony Watson, Joe Cokanasiga and Semesa Rokoduguni, all England internationals, in the backs. As if that wasn't enough, there's Scotland's Cameron Redpath and Fiji's Josh Matavesi.

But rugby players are like actors, in that even the best can look terrible if the production's not up to scratch. A script is just a script, it's not the law. That's why some of the best film directors are flexible, allow actors to ask questions and suggest changes during rehearsals – 'You know what, Marty? I reckon I should be saying this instead.' That's real collaboration, a director and his actors working together to make a film as good as possible. Sparkly, magical, different. But at Bath, we've got a director who wants to stick rigidly to the script, even though it's obvious the script isn't working.

There are occasional attempts at stirring speeches in training, but mostly the atmosphere is bleak, sometimes tragicomic. The attack coach's framework is ludicrously complicated. He's got two big boards with 30 or 40 principles on each. He divides his principles into different game models – 'If this kick happens, these five things might come into play. But if this kick happens, these five things might come into play', ad infinitum.

He's always asking, 'What's the game model if this happens?' The lads will all look blank, or stare at the ground, and he'll get annoyed, like a disappointed professor. I sometimes get the urge to speak up, but I know my words won't be well-received, because Neal doesn't really want me there, so I keep schtum instead. Sometimes, that feels nice, because it means avoiding conflict. But it can also be frustrating. I'll be sat there thinking, *Just keep it simple, mate. You only need four or five principles.*

We finally win a game in January, a one-point victory over Worcester. But I'm not involved again, after suffering another concussion against Northampton. Our attack coach gets sacked in mid-February, and they bring in a young academy coach called Ryan Davis, who I played with in the National Academy way back. I sit down with Ryan for a couple of hours, explain how I see the game, and he changes our training on the Monday. We then go four games unbeaten, and I can't help thinking, *If only we'd done this in pre-season.*

Neal sticks me on the bench for our European Champions Cup quarter-final against Edinburgh. *Fair enough*, I think, *Orlando is the future of the club, go for it.* But when it's still close with half an hour to go, it's screaming out for me to be introduced. Weirdly, Neal waits until Edinburgh have scored three more tries and only gives me 12 minutes.

A fortnight later, arch-rivals Gloucester pummel us 64–0, which is a performance directly related to the environment that's been created. A couple of fans have a go at me for smiling after the game, but what do they expect? Anyway, I've already told the club I'm leaving at the end of the season. To do what, I haven't yet decided.

Neal leaves me on the bench for the last two games of the season, at home against London Irish and away to Worcester. The old me would have reacted badly, because my sense of value would have been based on his decision not to play me. But the new me realises it doesn't really matter.

I head out with the boys after the Worcester game, which might have been my last in England had Neal played me. Anthony Watson says to me, 'Mate, I can't believe they didn't put you on.' I reply, 'There's no point being mad, Ant, that ain't gonna serve me going forward.'

It's been a terrible season on the pitch, with Bath finishing rock bottom of the table. There's no relegation, but it's still humiliating for such a famous old club. That said, it's been the most peaceful season I've ever had in rugby. It's also taught me that I'm no longer craving respect, that I'm just happy to be me. If the people in charge don't see me, so be it.

I prefer to focus on something Orlando says to me after our win over London Irish. 'Danny,' he says, 'I felt so good today, the freest I've ever felt on the field, and that's down to everything we've been working on in training.'

He's right, he was great in that game, but it had nothing to do with me. I'd given him a few pointers, to do with kicking and general understanding of the game, but he'd taken them on board and put them into action. That's what good coaching is, enabling players, rather than controlling them. And how beautiful it is to see players you've enabled go out and do their thing.

30

A HIGHER PLANE

Blackie's dead, and it's difficult to put into words how much I'll miss him. I'm angry with him – he spent his life making other people feel a million bucks and didn't look after his own health – but there's a lesson in that as well.

I'm so grateful that Blackie was part of my life. When I desperately needed someone to see, understand and love me, he was there, like a big, Geordie guardian angel. I'm not sure I'd be here now if it wasn't for Blackie. That's what Blackie did in a nutshell, get people who'd wandered off in the wrong direction back on track. I really do love that man.

On his birthday, I message his daughter, to ask how she's coping. She tells me she's finding things challenging but is managing to find some joy in life. When she asks how I am, I reply, 'Thanks to your dad, who convinced me to see myself for who I really am, rather than what other people were telling me I was, I'm in a far better place. I am love.'

That Blackie was able to connect with the old version of me and the old version of Jonny Wilkinson, two very different people on the face of it, is testament to what a great coach Blackie was. And I don't think it's an accident that as Blackie bows out, Jonny has become a special friend.

Me and Jonny hooked up again when I was getting ready to join Bath and have been training together for a year or so. But what started out as a couple of blokes just practising kicking has become something far deeper.

All that bitter rivalry stuff was concocted by the media. It made for a good story – squeaky clean Jonny versus bad boy Danny. Truth is, we always got on well enough, and we've been brought closer together by our beautiful relationships with Blackie.

Jonny's probably the most famous rugby player England has ever produced, the guy every kid wanted to be, but he's very humble. We trust each other, are able to be completely ourselves, which is probably why our conversation is so pure.

We normally start with an hour-long conversation to get into the flow, followed by some spectacular kicking. It's not like I turn up with a laminated agenda – *Today, the topics of conversation will be this, that and the other* – we just go wherever the conversation leads us. Nothing is off limits and there's no judgement.

We meet in a local park in Surrey, on a pitch so bad you wouldn't let an under-12 team play on it. Bald patches, dirty great holes, dog shit, you know the drill. To most people walking their pooches or pushing their kids on the swings, we're just a couple of mates kicking a ball to each other.

It's those long chats that enable us to execute our skills without even trying. I've got a great right foot, but I've gone through my entire career thinking my right foot is my 'wrong' foot, and my left foot is my 'right' one. But one session, I've got a tight quad in my left leg, so I kick with my right foot instead.

After a while, I'm not even watching where the ball is going. At one point, I reel off 10 kicks and Jonny says to me, 'Do you know where they ended up?' I tell him I don't, and he says, 'The first nine hit almost exactly the same spot on the wall and the last was just off.' That's because I was so in the present, ignoring limitations, and not paying any attention to the outcome.

My last game of rugby was for the Barbarians against Northampton on 26 November 2022. The fixture was a benefit for former Wasps and Worcester players, Worcester having been disbanded, Wasps having entered administration, been suspended from all rugby and relegated to the Championship. Now I've heard they're to be banished to the bottom of the league pyramid, which means they'll cease to be a professional outfit.

It really hurt when I heard about Wasps' plight. They're my childhood club and I've always had a strong affiliation with them. Wasps had a uniqueness that other clubs couldn't mimic. There was something beautiful about being part of a club that grew so many of its own players. I had team-mates from all walks of life, and the fanbase seemed to be more diverse than most. I always felt right at home at Wasps, whether that home was in west London,

High Wycombe or Coventry. Even the bad times at Wasps were perfect, because of what they taught me about life.

But it was obvious to anyone with half a brain that the finances in club rugby didn't add up, so I could see Wasps' collapse coming a mile off. There are lots of proud old clubs hanging on for dear life below the Premiership, and participation levels have plummeted at grassroots level. London Irish have followed Wasps and Worcester in going under, at the same time as other clubs, with wealthier owners, are talking about increasing the salary cap. Mindless.

I don't claim to have all the answers, but I've got a few suggestions. The biggest problem with English rugby is the product itself. Unlike football, which is constantly evolving, English rugby is averse to change, still clinging on to those same rugby 'values' from the 1950s. While football is rightly viewed as a game for everyone, English rugby is still viewed by many as a game for white middle-class people. Hardly anyone goes to private school, but half the England team did. I'm mixed-race and grew up on a council estate, but had I not got a scholarship to Whitgift, there's every chance I'd have been lost to another sport, probably football.

You can't really be having a go at private schools because English rugby would be in an even worse state without them. But imagine how much untapped talent there is in working-class communities. I'll sometimes watch basketball and think, *Imagine if some of these boys had played rugby instead, they'd be unstoppable.* I can only conclude the rugby authorities don't go looking, because it's not what they want their sport to look like. And if kids don't see themselves in a sport, they're unlikely to want to play it.

English cricket has some of the same problems as rugby, but at least it's tried to make itself more appealing to younger people. Some of the shots they play now – reverse slogs, ramp shots, one-handed pulls – would have made the 'it's just not cricket' brigade tut-tut 20 years ago, but now they're the norm. Modern cricket is all about expressing yourself, trying to make the crowd gasp, and not worrying about messing up and making the crowd jeer instead.

I like that famous quote by the Trinidadian writer CLR James: 'What do they know of cricket who only cricket know?' You can apply that to English rugby, which is mostly run by people who look, sound and think the same, because they mostly come from the same traditional rugby backgrounds.

It's like a big company with 15 board members who all went to Oxford or Cambridge. When that company has a board meeting, how many ideas are in the room? One, because those 15 board members all think the same.

When Eddie came out with that statement about private schools churning out players who can't think for themselves, he was onto something. The irony being, he hasn't created an England environment in which players can think for themselves, with game scenarios and decision-making drills.

Eddie's always going on about the importance of leadership, but the only leaders he's interested in are people who see the game the same as him. Meanwhile, any player who thinks differently to Eddie, and lets him know about it, is soon bombed out. That's why most England players put up and shut up, because the badge, the status and the money are more important to them than the truth. Then again, I was no different, at least under Lanny and Eddie, so I can't exactly have a go at anyone else for their lack of integrity.

Kids nowadays don't just want to be told what to do, they want to have fun, work things out for themselves, express themselves, be themselves. That requires coaches to be open-minded, compassionate. And by loosening things up, more kids will want to play the game, they'll want to play the game better, more people will want to watch it, and England will have more success.

As it is, even if a kid attains some success by being true to himself and unconventional, the messages will suddenly change when he starts playing professionally. Instead of thinking, *Wow, this kid's got something different, let's try to figure out why he sees what he sees and maybe it will help the team*, his coaches will want him to be like everyone else. That means he's just doing what he's told, even if it doesn't feel right. And he's no longer playing for the sheer joy of it, which is what made him so special in the first place.

The two best coaches I've played under are Brian Ashton and Shaun Edwards, but Brian got binned by England because he was too romantic and idealist – 'English rugby can't be played that way!' – and Shaun has never been given the opportunity, despite doing great things with Wales and France.

One thing they have in common is not thinking they know everything about the game. They leave lots of room for manoeuvre, are big on instinct and encouraging players to come up with their own answers. Their training isn't solely geared towards winning games of rugby because they understand that winning or losing can't be your main motivation if you want to evolve. And if you train without outcomes in mind, you'll play in the moment, with more freedom and intuition, and you'll naturally win more games than you lose.

How ironic that two of the best coaches in the game right now are Stuart Lancaster and Andy Farrell, who have both worked wonders in Ireland. Since Lanny joined Leinster in 2016, they've won the Champions Cup once and been runners-up twice, while Andy's Ireland team is one of the best in the world.

Before Ireland's Grand Slam game against England in 2023, an interviewer asked Andy if his players were feeling the pressure. Andy replied, 'No, it's just a game of rugby. The boys will handle it.' That's how to get your team playing thinking rugby, rather than doing everything at 100 mph.

Andy's made Ireland formidable by increasing their game understanding, particularly when it comes to tempo. Every team should want their players to have as much thinking time as possible, and by the time Ireland's backs have reached the line, they're usually ready to make the right decision. Changing to that mindset from a traditional phase to phase attack isn't easy and is testament to Andy's rugby intelligence and coaching ability.

English rugby is still miles ahead of every other country in terms of cash and playing numbers, but the national side has had one short period of dominance in the professional era. Since winning the World Cup in 2003, it's mostly been a tale of underachievement. Not even exciting underachievement.

Eddie was in charge for seven years, during which time I saw England overwhelm decent teams maybe two or three times, which you then have to call anomalies. That's because professionalism in English rugby has meant rigidity and uniformity. It's meant coaches springing up all over the place telling people how rugby *should be*, training the life out of players and programming them with statistics.

Rugby is a simple game, it's only made complicated, from grassroots to the elite level, by coaches who want to justify their initialled tracksuits. But too many of those coaches don't really understand the game – how to manipulate defenders, pull them out of position, create numbers in attack, attack space. So while games like football and basketball have developed tactically over the years, rugby looks much the same as it did 20 years ago – except maybe more rigid.

There's a reason Sam Allardyce doesn't coach in the Premier League anymore, namely because his methods went out of fashion and were no longer winning football matches. But there are still a lot of Allardyce types in English rugby, because you can still win games playing Allardyce-type rugby.

Having been optimistic that at least the England team might start playing some decent rugby after Eddie's sacking and Steve Borthwick's appointment, now I'm not sure. Look at what happened to Marcus Smith when Borthers picked him to start at 10 against France in the Six Nations: England got drubbed 53–10 at Twickenham and Marcus got hammered in the press.

But there's almost nothing Marcus could have done to prevent that from happening, because England's pack got demolished and he was living off scraps. When he did get the ball, his team-mates weren't in the right positions, so the only thing he could have done different was kick more.

But instead of working with Marcus, getting him to understand that he needs to go into every game knowing exactly where his team-mates are at any given moment, they axed him for the next fixture against Ireland. Meanwhile, people on social media were saying England need to be grittier, tougher, nastier. I thought, *Getting grittier, tougher and nastier always seems to be the answer to English rugby's problems. What about getting more skilful?*

Marcus is still young, has great footwork and can beat defenders for fun. If he can improve his reading of the game and decision-making, he could win far more caps than me. But I suspect England in the short-term are going to be very stats-driven, with an awful lot of kicking, and not a lot of fun to watch.

In stark contrast, I'd love rugby to be thought of as a beautiful, artistic game that kids watch on TV and nag their parents to play, instead of thinking it's boring and impossible to understand. I'd like them to think rugby is fun, exciting, a game for thinkers and non-conformists.

And I'd like people who have followed rugby union for years to realise it can be played differently, that physicality isn't the be all and end all, that it can exist on a higher plane.

Things have to change, because if people carry on telling themselves that rugby is wonderful as it is, it will be a niche interest within a decade.

Epilogue

JUST BEING

I almost forgot to mention – I'm a grandfather! How surreal is that? But I absolutely love it, even the inevitable gags about sitting in front of the fire with a blanket over my knees while sucking on a Werther's Original.

Rosie, who's my stepdaughter's daughter, calls me 'Pops'. Whenever I say goodbye to her, she cries and holds her arms out, because she doesn't want me to go. And I always make sure I let her know that I'm coming back.

Rosie, who's seven, and her sister Lily, who's one, are bundles of energy and full of love. I'm so looking forward to seeing them blossom into the wonderful women I know they're going to be. I'd do anything for them, as I would for their mum Jade and Victoria's son Kam. I love them all as if they were my own.

If you'd said to a 10-year-old me, 'You're going to have a beautiful family with three kids and two grandkids', I'd have been the happiest boy in the world. Throw in all my uncles, aunties and cousins in Trinidad and Tobago (I'm especially close to my cousin Trisha, who I love dearly), and I've got it pretty good. It's not what you'd call a traditional family, but traditional families aren't always what they're cracked up to be.

A guy I know, a famous sportsman, has convinced himself he needs to be having sex with as many women as possible, because that suits his 'lion-like' personality. But now I'm married to Victoria, I'm not having to control anything. We were recently in a restaurant and Victoria was convinced the waitresses were trying to hit on me, but I honestly didn't notice. I'd never go back to that way of being – hoovering up crumbs of short-term pleasure, simply because I couldn't stand sitting with my own thoughts – because I remember how horrible it made me feel in the long run.

I play nine-a-side every Monday, and it always runs 10 or 15 minutes over. The other day I was shouting, 'Lads, I wanna go home to my missus, stop avoiding your wives!' One of them shot back with, 'Dan, wait 'til you've been married as long as I have, you'd rather shag one of us lot.' I understood where he was coming from, because I've been there. But not with Victoria.

After my England dream was torpedoed in 2019, I spent a lot of time drifting, until Victoria spotted me flailing and scooped me up. We both could have chosen an easier route to love, but it wouldn't have been as real.

Before I met Victoria, I didn't know how to give my heart to a woman. I now know that's because I was looking for love in all the wrong places, and that it actually springs from within. Victoria was the first person in my life I'd been completely honest with. A lot of what I told her wasn't pretty, but she showed me so much compassion and kindness. And I had renewed hope, because she was bringing our child into the world.

We're still ironing little bits out, but any good relationship is an ongoing project. And we're in a beautiful place together. When I'm out and about, I miss Victoria, can't wait to get home and find out how she's doing. And I love going to bed with her every night and waking up with her every morning. She is, without a doubt, the most incredible person I've ever met.

I haven't retired from rugby – even the word 'retired' makes me wince – and if the right team wants me to play for them, and it sounds exciting, I'll do it.

As I've said, my last game was for the Barbarians against Northampton in November 2022. We had a load of Wasps players in our line-up, blokes who had recently been made redundant, and we all sang Adele's 'Someone Like You' in the changing room beforehand, which was better than most motivational speeches I've heard down the years.

Most of the lads started out timid but everyone was roaring by the end. So many retired rugby players tell me how little of their careers they enjoyed, because there was far too much rigidity, anxiety, grind and tedium, so it was refreshing to feel that freedom and looseness.

I've had offers to play in Japan, and they're very tempting. It's decent money and I like the idea of living a beautiful life somewhere exotic.

Quade Cooper messaged me recently: 'Mate, you can't hang your boots up. Come over to Japan and play with me. You'll earn a fortune and have a great time.' I tell him

I haven't hung my boots up, but when I dig into the details, none of the offers feels right. It's me just scratching an itch, thinking I've still got stuff to prove. And I wouldn't be helping anyone by heading off to Japan.

If I play rugby again, great. Everywhere I've been, whether it was at a club which was expected to win things, or a club where I had to run things on the back foot in order to achieve some success, I've transformed things and made people around me see the game in a different light. With my head as it is now, and in an open and honest environment, I think I'd love it, because I'd just be living it.

If not, no problem. It's time to start looking at the bigger picture and getting in the groove for however many years I've got left. I've learned to live my life the way I play rugby – reacting to what's in front of me, not grasping at the past. Because when you're fully engaged in the moment, you get freedom and spontaneity. You're still going to make mistakes, which you need to take responsibility for, but you're coming from a place of purity, being true to yourself and not just playing the game.

People will be reading this and thinking, *How did not playing the game work out for your rugby career, Danny?* They'd be right, not playing the game made it far more onerous and uncomfortable than it could have been. But I can look in the mirror and say, *Mate, at least you weren't trying to be something you weren't just to fit in; you had integrity and stood up for what you really believed in.*

There are plenty of less talented English players than me with more international caps. And I used to wonder what the last however many years might have looked like for England had a coach given me a run in the team and licence to lead the team through responsibility, accountability, freedom, honesty and love. I suspect we'd have won more games and played far more attractive rugby – and Twickenham would have been a lot noisier. I'd have got that team playing some crowd-pleasing tunes.

Not getting picked for the 2019 World Cup broke me and doused my passion, I just didn't know it back then. It was only when I started writing about it that the tears came. I stood up for what I felt was best for the team and players in every environment. I was targeted and ostracised because I felt differently and thought differently to most coaches. I was feared and spoken about as if I was the worst kind of character, simply because I challenged the hierarchy and traditional way of doing things. I was publicly dismissed by coaches. And I could never respond as I was relentlessly pursuing my dream of playing for England.

God knows I didn't make things easy for myself. I used to look back and think, *Why did you behave like that? Why didn't you try to fix things sooner?* But they're pointless questions, because I was a different person then, with seemingly unshakeable needs and desires. And the only way to let go of mistakes is to be accountable, recognise the behaviour and where it came from, and forgive yourself. That allows you to sit in the present, which is a far more peaceful place to be than wallowing in chaos from the past.

Spending so much time going out of my mind because I couldn't get what I wanted, taking painkillers to block out the feelings of being misunderstood, and desperately trying to understand myself, forced me to examine those needs and desires. Now I realise that so much of my craving, in rugby and in my relationships with women, was my ego working overtime, and me desperately searching for validation and wanting to feel enough.

I was a kid with an innocent love for sport. The sporting arena was my happy place, my freedom. If as a seven-year-old I had the choice of a maths class or a sports field, I chose the sports field, because it lit up my soul. It's why I went to Whitgift, because I wanted to play rugby with my two best mates, Neville and Adam, who felt more like brothers.

Then when I started getting paid and forensically judged for my efforts, on and off the pitch, I was constantly thinking, *Am I enough?* I focused on the external, on what people were saying about me, based on snippets of my life. At times, it was very hard to stay strong and remember who I really was. Luckily, I managed to reconnect with my youthful passion. I remembered that my talent was God given, not something I created. As such, I was able to relinquish the notion that I made things happen on a rugby pitch, and that I should be proud or ashamed of my efforts. But I am proud of standing up for what I believed in.

If you allow yourself to be defined by what you achieved in the past, you'll find it difficult to thrive in the present. It's like that old phrase, 'You're only as good as the last good thing you did.' That's not ideal if the last good thing you did was play well in a game that almost everyone else has forgotten.

* * *

Constantly feeling rejected by my mum and abandoned by my dad was obviously tough, and created so many difficulties for me as an adult, but I love them both dearly and unconditionally and have no ill feelings towards them. Why would I? Paradoxically, they were my biggest catalysts to transform myself, to heal and let go. Everything I've needed to thrive in this world I got from them.

Dad's absence affected how I interacted with authority figures all the way through my career, and I accept that I gave too many coaches reasons to judge me. But it also meant I've had to figure things out for myself. That's what made me the player I was and why I'm now more curious about life than most, doing things that inspire me and take me out of my comfort zone.

Mum loved me when I was a kid, and I'm sure she thought she was showing it. But because of her life experiences, her way of showing love didn't involve kind words or affection. That lack of obvious love and, at times, respect, meant I treated women like a child with his toys, to be picked up and put down on a whim. And so often my relationships ended in traumatic fashion. I was emotionally unavailable. But Mum taught me that you have to confront yourself if you want normal, healthy relationships, which is what I have now with Victoria and the kids.

Mum definitely softened after her stroke. Now she's decided to return to her own home, we'll pay her a visit and she'll barely say a word to me. But it doesn't make me bitter or angry or sad, and I'll keep turning up. Not because I want to make up for the feelings of rejection or dismissal I felt my whole life, but because I want her to live the best life she can.

My whole career, people have been telling me who I am and why I don't fit in. Sometimes, it's been like living in an alternative reality, in which strangers know me better than I know myself. There was a cacophony of voices in my head, and the only time I could find peace was when I stepped onto a rugby field and did what I do best. All that abuse could have ended very badly for me, as it did for Caroline. There was a point when I didn't want to be here, and when Caroline took her own life, it felt like everything inside of me had broken.

I've had to dig deep, my survival depended on it. In doing so, I've uncovered so much about myself that otherwise would have remained buried. And while I haven't gaslit myself into believing I've loved every minute of my rugby career, and I've never felt entirely welcome in the so-called rugby family, I better appreciate how fortunate I was to be born with a gift to play sport and make it my living. And I'd love everyone to know what it feels like to be at the levers of a team that's working perfectly. It really is beautiful.

I loved all the teams I've played for and so many of the people I've met through rugby. I know a lot of them felt, and continue to feel, the same constraints as I did, but they still found time to show me love and support throughout my career, for which I'm incredibly thankful.

When you've been dismissed by a coach, because they fear what you might do, even though you only ever wanted what was best for the team, it can feel like the end of the world. When people who can't do what you can do are playing ahead of you, it can feel like you're the victim of a great injustice. When the media pulls out another dodgy story, just when you're on the verge of England selection, those feelings of victimhood can be so intense that they seem inescapable. But no-one has a perfect life, no-one gets everything they want. And following your passion isn't meant to be a smooth, uneventful ride, it's meant to be an all-terrain epic, taking in success, failure, acceptance, rejection, and much more besides. Your route might not be as chaotic as mine, but at least you know it can be.

The one thing that connects us all is suffering, and I'm grateful for everything that's happened in my life, because it's how I managed to figure out what I needed to know about myself. And it was those moments that almost ground me into dust that were most valuable, in terms of my long-term growth. If you take the time to understand the rough stretches, you can make them work for you. I can't feel the sting of rejection or failure anymore, I don't care about being judged or misunderstood, because they're all things that led me here now, which is a place full of love and compassion.

In the same way, it makes no sense to harbour ill-feeling towards anyone I haven't seen eye to eye with during my rugby career. Who wants to be an old man who's bitter and angry at the world? Like Grampa Simpson, shaking his fist and yelling at clouds. Not me, not anyone. But you don't become a chilled, smiley, white-haired dude by accident. You only discover that love, compassion and understanding are the answer by going on a journey of self-discovery. Also on that journey, you'll learn that by judging others, you're harming yourself. You have to clean stuff up, let go of things, come to terms with the fact that money and status, and selling yourself out to get both, don't make you happy.

My timing was always one of my main attributes on a rugby field, but it could be diabolical off it, like when I got done for drink-driving straight after a man-of-the-match performance for England or arrested before I'd played a competitive game for Gloucester. It didn't help that the tabloids were hounding me, or that I had a girlfriend who kept telling them where I was, but still, I gave people too many excuses to write me off as a bit of a dickhead.

But in terms of the right characters coming into my life at the right moment, I was blessed. People who quite easily could have been just someone else's parent, or just a teacher, coach or physio, decided to be much more than that. When I hooked up with Blackie, I started looking outside of myself, while also gaining a broader perspective from a variety of enlightened people – including spiritual gurus, stoics and scientists – or anyone whose thoughts resonated with me, and made it easier to deal with what was going on inside. Then I became closer to Jonny, who happened to be on a similar journey to me, before Victoria popped up and saved me from drowning. Writing this book has been a great privilege, especially as at one point I didn't think I'd be around to tell my story. Every time I became emotional, I was thankful, because I knew that was trauma I hadn't addressed leaving my body.

Faith has allowed me to build trust in myself. Whenever a negative thought arises, instead of it taking over my mind and body, as when I was a child or at my lowest ebb, I have faith that love will take care of it. And I know that once the thought is gone, joy and beauty will replace it. Instead, I'm comforted by knowing that beauty will spring from them, like flowers from the ground.

Everyone is born with magic inside of them, but loss, failure, rejection, abandonment and other bad things happen, and the mind gets filled with negative chatter. I got distracted by misplaced desires and material things. I tried to replace the emptiness I felt by wanting to be seen as the best. The good news is, I'm living proof that it's possible to salvage the magic.

Now that I know and love myself, and how I feel is entirely down to me, I can be the architect of my own future. I'm excited about what's to come, even though I don't know what it will look like. If and when I feel compelled to do something, I'll just know it's right.

I feel like the Danny my mates knew when we were kids. Exuberant, unafraid, free, full of running. Still not playing the game by anyone else's rules.

ACKNOWLEDGEMENTS

I'd like to thank Ben Dirs for making it really easy to talk to him. We spent hours upon hours together and he really put in the effort for this project. Very grateful. I'd like to thank HarperCollins and the team, as everyone I met was warm, friendly and engaging. I'd like to thank Adam Humphrey for always wearing your heart on your sleeve and bringing the energy every time. I'd like to thank my old agent and friend Olly for being there with me through many uncomfortable moments, as well as a thank you to Rhodri and his team at Footprint for the hours of work and dedication they've put in, and for instilling belief and confidence the whole way.

I would like to thank Mr O'D, you were the first coach who really believed in me and made me feel special. I would like to thank Roger Hamilton Brown for seeing something in me and taking me to Rosslyn Park when I was 10! I'd like to thank all my Rosslyn Park coaches, Tony Durrant, Steve Poole, Phil Stringer and more I haven't mentioned for letting me be me when sometimes you may have wanted to wring my neck. To all my Rosslyn

Park team-mates, those were the days, we had so much fun and won a couple games along the way. To Neville, Ed, Dom, I'll always appreciate you all, felt more like brothers. To Alun Powell, Rob Smith, thank you for those academy sessions back in the day, they really set me up for my career. I'd like to thank Dr Barnett, you always looked after me at school, your vision to help your students prosper, especially the ones that could have been troublesome with a little talent, is felt by many! I'd like to thank Shaun Edwards for the countless hours, care and compassion and friendship you showed me. Forever grateful. I'd like to thank Brian Ashton, for stimulating and challenging my ideas and beliefs, allowing me to constantly evolve on the field. I'd like to thank Luke, Mel Izak and Cruzie for showing me the beauty of how a family operates. I'd like to thank Laird, Gabby, Reece, Brody for always making me feel welcome and taking me into your inner circle and showing me the love you did, as well as introducing me to the OGs Hutch, Darin and the crew as well as my bro Joakim. We could all do with a James Williams in our lives. Thank you mate for being you and taking me down to Malibu. I'd like to thank Malcolm Farquharson for always telling it to me straight, showing me love and looking out for me. I'd like to thank Kevin Lidlow, for always taking care of my body, mind and soul. You are an angel in human form, you conduct yourself with such humility yet are the very best in the game. I'd like to thank Blackie because I know he is reading this and is with me, thank you for truly seeing me at a time when no one else did. Thank you for igniting the spark within me again, thank you for showing me it's okay to lead with your heart. Thank you for connecting Jonny and myself, as I have a feeling you're always listening to our conversations and smiling. I'd like to thank Margot Wells, not only the greatest fitness coach but also a great friend whose support and love have been humbling. I'd like to thank all my teammates I've played with, I've enjoyed you all one way or another. Special shout out to the 'Brothers' – Nathan, Willie, Christian, Juan, Marcus, Gaby, Ashley, Nizaam, Kurtley, Kyle, Antonio, that was a fun two years among the chaos. I'd like to thank my Trini family, I love you all and look forward to liming in the future. I'd like to thank Trisha for always seeing my heart and seeing me. I'd like to thank Jade, Kameron, Rosie Q and Lily for filling my days with laughter, joy and school runs. As well as Stepdad/Grandad duties which I love. I'd like to thank Mum for the lessons and her commitment early on, thank you for showing me how to be resilient and never give up. I'd like to thank Dad for brightening up my younger years and introducing me to sport. I'd also like to thank the media for holding me accountable. I just hope one day, you start doing that to yourselves with how you speak about people and the effect you have not only on them but the readers too and the younger population, who think it's okay to judge and critique in the same way you do. By being conscious of the way you write, you will uplift this whole country rather than keep a grey cloud over it. I have faith it will change in the near future ... God is love.

PICTURE CREDITS

While every effort has been made to trace the owners of copyright material reproduced herein and secure permissions, the publishers would like to apologise for any omissions and will be pleased to incorporate missing acknowledgements in any future edition of this book.

p1, p7 (bottom right), p8 (top left, bottom) courtesy the author
p1 (bottom right), p2, p3 (top, bottom), p4 (bottom right), p6 (bottom), p8 (top, middle) David Rogers/Getty Images
p3 (middle), p4 (bottom right) David Davies/PA Images/Alamy Stock Photo
p4 (top) Ian Kington/AFP via Getty Images
p4 (bottom left) Allstar Picture Library Ltd/Alamy Stock Photo
p5 (top) WENN Rights Ltd/Alamy Stock Photo
p5 (bottom) Scott Barbour/Getty Images
p6 (top) Graham Chadwick/ANL/Shutterstock.com
p7 (top left) Dave Thompson/Getty Images
p7 (top right) Dominic Lipinski/PA Images/Alamy Stock Photo
p7 (bottom left) Mike Egerton/PA Images/Alamy Stock Photo

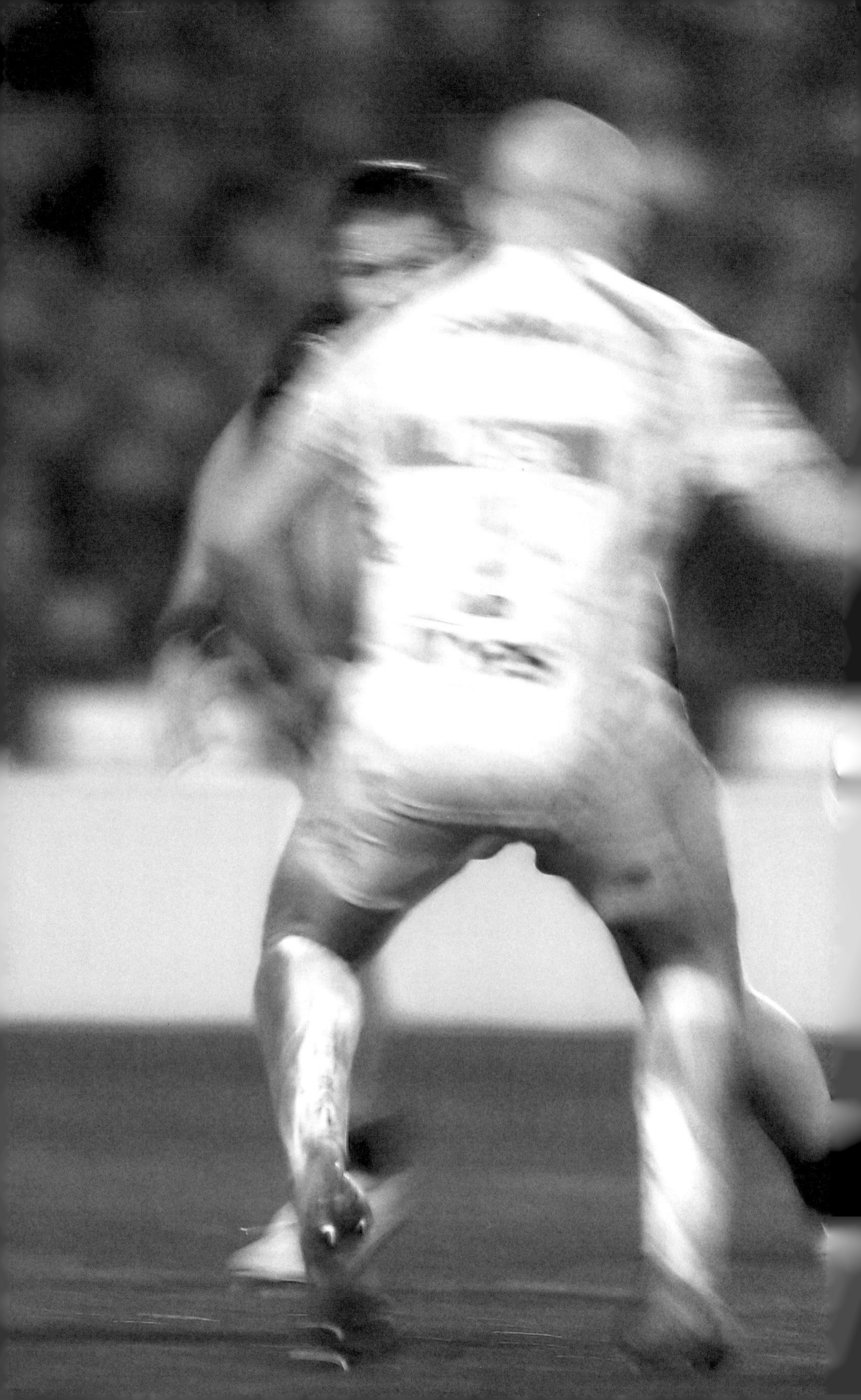